Yoga Beats Asthma

To Desi Luckhoo-Hachiya, with much love and gratitude

Yoga Beats Asthma

Simple exercises and breathing techniques
to relieve asthma and respiratory disorders

Stella Weller

With a foreword by Marie E. Faughnan, M.D., F.R.C.P.C.
Division of Respiratory Medicine, St Michael's Hospital, Toronto

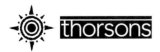

Thorsons
An Imprint of HarperCollins*Publishers*
77–85 Fulham Palace Road,
Hammersmith, London W6 8JB

The website address is: www.thorsonselement.com

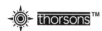

and *Thorsons* are trademarks of
HarperCollins*Publishers* Limited

First published 2003

10 9 8 7 6 5 4 3 2 1

Photography by Guy Hearn
Text illustrations by Peter Cox Associates

A catalogue record for this book
is available from the British Library

ISBN 0 00 715449 6

Printed and bound in Great Britain by
Scotprint, Haddington, East Lothian

Contents

Acknowledgments

I thank everyone who has in any way contributed to this work. I am particularly grateful to Wanda Whiteley, Susanna Abbott, Natasha Fidler, Gigi Bettencourt-Gomes, Fela Adeyemi and other members of the editorial team at HarperCollins: Simon Gerratt, Paul Redhead, Kate Latham, Barbara Vesey.

To Linda Howard, Jane Kupfer and Debra Nelson, three outstanding librarians.

To Marie E. Faughnan, MD, FRCPC, for reading the manuscript, writing the Foreword, and offering several very useful suggestions.

To Nadia Knarr, for her kind assistance in painstakingly reading the manuscript.

Special thanks go to Walter, David, Karl and Lora for their constant love, encouragement and support.

In the last 15 years, we have seen considerable progress in the treatment of asthma. A more sophisticated understanding of the disease has led to improved medical therapy. Physicians and scientists agree that asthma is an inflammatory disease, and therefore anti-inflammatory medications are the cornerstone of medical treatment.

Unfortunately, the last 15 years have also seen an increase in the prevalence and severity of asthma, especially in the inner city and in developing countries. This is likely due to increased allergens and irritants in our indoor and outdoor environments. Treating asthma, therefore, is not just about improving an asthmatic's response to the environment, but it also involves improving the asthmatic's environment itself.

While many patients still require medications to control this disease, doctors can also advise their patients about ways to reduce allergens and irritants in the home and work environments. These changes can include saying goodbye to the beloved cat, cutting down on dust mites in the bedroom and moving smokers out of the house and workplace.

Although anti-inflammatory medications, predominantly inhaled corticosteroids, are the mainstay of therapy, and environmental clean-ups help tremendously, the effects of both are further complemented by other non-medical approaches. For instance, stress can be an important trigger for asthma symptoms, but stress management tends to be neglected in asthma treatment. Finding the time and the right method for reducing stress can be a challenge for people who do not know where to turn for this kind of help. Stella Weller gives asthma sufferers a practical approach to managing stress and its effect on breathing. As part of a full complement of asthma therapy, Weller introduces yoga into the mix. Yoga helps the practitioner relax and breathe.

What makes Weller's book particularly valuable to asthma sufferers is its two-fold approach: The first half of the book presents an extensive account of asthma – its symptoms, various treatments and their side-effects. The second half of the book offers detailed descriptions of specific yoga exercises. Recent clinical studies have shown that yoga can improve symptoms in the asthmatic. While Weller does not suggest that yoga replace medical treatment or the advice of a physician, she directs readers to the benefits of yoga as an effective component in a full complement of asthma treatments.

People who want to know more about asthma and what they can do to feel better will find Weller's book a valuable resource.

MARIE E. FAUGHNAN MD FRCPC
DIVISION OF RESPIRATORY MEDICINE, ST. MICHAEL'S HOSPITAL
ASSISTANT PROFESSOR, UNIVERSITY OF TORONTO

List of Illustrations

Yoga Postures and Breathing Exercises Suitable for Children

Balance Postures (to promote steadiness and calm):

Breathing Exercises (an important tool to help in coping with anxiety states and difficult breathing):

Important Note

This book is not intended to take the place of medical advice from a qualified doctor. We recommend that readers who are interested in natural approaches to controlling asthma seek the advice and guidance of a trained health professional before implementing any of the suggestions in this book. Neither the publisher nor the author takes any responsibility for any action, activity or administration of medicine or preparation by anyone reading or following the information in this book.

Introduction

Despite remarkable advances in technology and a significant increase in general knowledge about asthma, the incidence of this breathing disorder, and deaths therefrom, have risen sharply since the mid-1980s.

Asthma affects nearly 100 million people worldwide. It is estimated that 17 million Americans suffer from the disorder, making it the most chronic illness in adults and children, with 15 million physician visits a year and 10 million missed days from school. More than three million people in the U.K. suffer from it, and it causes approximately 2,000 deaths a year. Annual prescriptions for asthma treatments in Britain almost doubled between 1982 and 1991, with N.H.S. (National Health Service) costs rocketing from £50 million to £350 million in that period of time. Surveys also indicate that asthma has doubled during the past 20 years in Australia and New Zealand.

The prospects for asthma sufferers and their families is far from dismal, however. With appropriate education and a guided plan of management, asthma sufferers can be taught the skillful use of tools they already have with and within themselves to control this treatable condition. And there is perhaps no more fulfilling experience for a healer than to see someone – often a child – go from exclusive dependence on powerful drugs to greater reliance on his or her own natural powers of breathing and other personal resources.

The consensus among medical professionals is that asthma is an inflammatory

condition of the airways which limits airflow to the lungs and which produces a
disturbance in the normal pattern of breathing. This points researchers and therapists
in four fruitful directions:

1. Avoiding or reducing the stressors that trigger asthma
2. Correcting the breathing pattern and restoring efficient breathing
3. Undoing various muscular tensions by developing awareness and promoting relaxation
4. Managing the emotions associated with asthma episodes, so as to gain a feeling of control and of confidence, and consequently a greatly enhanced sense of well-being.

Yoga Beats Asthma sheds light, in reader-friendly language, on this reversible
condition of the airways with its variable airflow limitation and hyper-responsiveness
to various stimuli. This book also discusses various related topics, including:

- asthma symptoms and what produces them
- risk factors
- triggers
- medicines and other treatments in current use
- preventive measures
- suitable exercise
- nutrition
- voluntary controlled respiration to help you use your breathing apparatus to the fullest advantage and to allay the anxiety that often accompanies asthma.

Research-based support for the use of breathing techniques for coping with various
respiratory and emotional difficulties continues to grow. Organizations devoted to
teaching people how to make the best use of their respiratory resources are also on
the increase. But the power of the breath and of exercises providing support to the
respiratory system have long been known to the practitioners of yoga. *Yoga Beats
Asthma*, as an ideal companion to orthodox medical treatments, beautifully utilizes
this centuries-old wisdom by integrating technological advances with skills that
empower people to make choices and feel a sense of control over their lives.

Your Breathing System

Understanding asthma is helped by first understanding your breathing (respiratory) system, so in this chapter we'll take a look at how this system works.

Nasal Matters

Your nose is much more than just an appendage on your face and a portal for the entry of air into the body. In fact, specialists in diseases of the nose (rhinologists) can list more than two dozen functions that the nose performs. These include: filtering, warming, and moisturizing inhaled air; directing air flow; bringing in oxygen; registering the sense of smell; creating mucus (a viscous fluid secreted by the mucous membranes); providing a channel for drainage of the sinuses, and interacting with the nervous system.

Fig. 1. Section of the face and neck, showing the upper respiratory passages

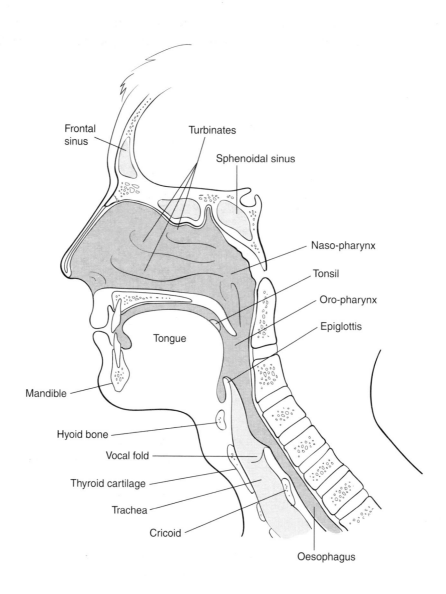

THE SINUSES

The sinuses are hollow spaces in the skull that open into the nose. Although their function is not fully understood, it is known that, in part, they lend resonance to the voice.

Fig. 2. The sinuses

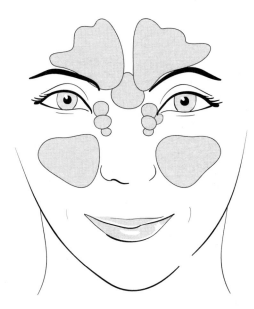

The cells lining the sinuses produce mucus, which traps particles and bacteria. Cilia, which are tiny, hairlike projections (see page 5), clear mucus and debris from the sinuses into the nose, and from there into the mouth or throat. When the opening of a sinus is blocked, mucus accumulates and bacteria thrive in it. This can result in infection.

A sinus infection can precipitate an asthma episode. It can also cause you to be more sensitive to other asthma triggers and make asthma resistant to treatment until the infection is cleared.

One way of helping to prevent blocked passageways, and infections such as sinusitis, is the regular practice of a technique called *neti,* or the nasal wash, which is described on page 125.

THE TURBINATES

Within the nasal cavity are three seashell-like bulges called turbinates. They stir and circulate air entering the nose, so that it passes over a much greater surface area. Too much turbulence, however, may cause breathing difficulties. This depends more on the arrangement of the turbinates and other structures than on the actual size of the passageways themselves.

Fig. 3. Cross-section of the nasal cavity showing the turbinates

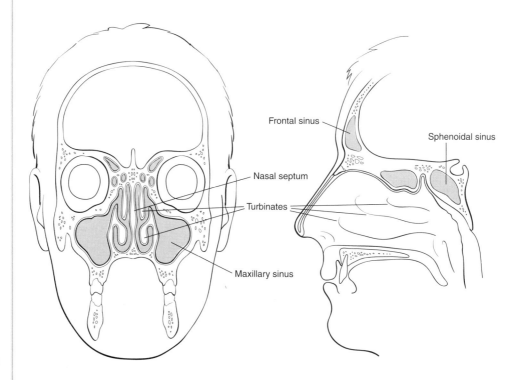

MUCUS BLANKET

The inside of the nose is lined with a mucous membrane that has the special property of being able to secrete mucus. Mucus picks up and carries away dust and other particles, various forms of debris, microbes such as bacteria, viruses and fungi, and other foreign agents that can invade delicate nasal tissues and cause infection.

Mucus is in constant motion, carrying along everything it has trapped, in a sort of 'mucus blanket'. The movement of this 'blanket' is the work of millions of tiny hairlike structures called cilia, which grow out of the mucous membrane.

CILIA

Cilia move back and forth about 12 times per second, 24 hours a day, in a well-coordinated wave-like fashion. They waft mucus along the throat, where it is either coughed up, sneezed out or swallowed and passed into the intestinal tract, where digestive enzymes dissolve it and its contents.

In a healthy body, this system works beautifully, but it understandably breaks down when certain respiratory disorders exist. Interestingly, after you have smoked only one cigarette, the cilia are paralysed for about an hour and a half. Habitual smoking eventually causes permanent paralysis of these hairlike structures. In addition, ciliary action is affected by alcohol, which diminishes mucus clearance from the lungs. Absence of moisture for even a few minutes can also destroy the delicate cilia.

Respiratory Structures

In addition to the nose, the structures of the respiratory system include: the pharynx (throat), which communicates with the larynx (voice box), and the esophagus (food-pipe) behind. The larynx is continuous with the pharynx above, and opens into the trachea (windpipe) below. (Part of the larynx can be seen as a protrusion at the front of the neck, known as the Adam's apple.)

THE BRONCHIAL TREE

Think of your respiratory system as an upside-down tree minus the roots. The trachea, which is at the top, may be considered the trunk. It divides into two main branches called bronchi (singular: bronchus). These are air passages which divide into smaller lobar and segmental bronchi, which in turn branch into smaller structures (bronchioles), of which there are about eight million. They terminate in alveoli (air sacs; singular: alveolus) where an exchange of gases occurs (see the section on gas exchange, page 12). Think of these as the leaves of this imaginary upside-down tree. It is estimated that there are 24 million alveoli at birth; by the time you are eight years old you have the adult number of 300 million.

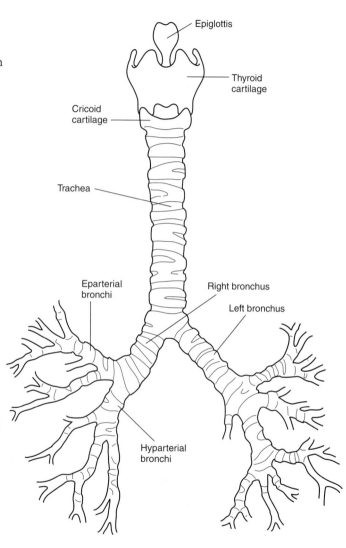

Fig. 4. The bronchial tree, showing the trachea, bronchi, bronchioles and alveoli

Epiglottis

Thyroid cartilage

Cricoid cartilage

Trachea

Eparterial bronchi

Right bronchus

Left bronchus

Hyparterial bronchi

The Lungs

The two lungs are the principal organs of respiration. They are located in the chest cavity, one each side separated by the heart and its great blood vessels and by other vital structures.

The lungs are cone-shaped, with the narrower part (apex) at the top. Their base rests on the diaphragm (see page 10); their outer surface is in contact with the ribs, and their posterior (rear) border is in contact with the spine.

The right lung consists of three lobes, but the left lung has only two, to accommodate the heart, which fits snugly between the two lungs, lying mainly in a hollow next to the left lung.

Each lobe of the lungs is composed of smaller divisions called lobules. A small bronchial tube enters each lobule, and as it divides and subdivides, its walls become thinner, finally ending in air sacs.

Fig. 5. Lungs and air passages. Insert shows alveoli at the end of the air passages

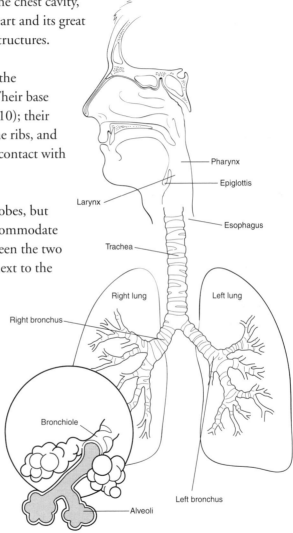

Pharynx

Epiglottis

Larynx

Esophagus

Trachea

Right lung

Left lung

Right bronchus

Bronchiole

Left bronchus

Alveoli

Lung tissue is elastic, porous, and spongy, and is capable of floating in water because of the air it contains.

The primary purpose of the lungs is to bring air and blood together so that oxygen can be transported to the blood and carbon dioxide removed from the blood.

BLOOD VESSELS OF THE LUNGS

The pulmonary (lung) artery carries deoxygenated (oxygen-poor) blood from the right side of the heart into the lungs for oxygenation. The pulmonary veins then return oxygenated (oxygen-rich) blood to the left side of the heart for distribution all over the body. Pulmonary circulation is unusual: in most cases throughout the body, arteries usually carry oxygenated blood, and veins carry deoxygenated blood. With the blood vessels of the lungs, the opposite is true.

PLEURA

Each lung is surrounded by a double layer of membrane known as pleura. The pulmonary pleura closely invests (surrounds) the lungs and separates its lobes. It is then reflected at the root of the lungs and forms the parietal (wall) pleura, which covers the interior chest wall and the thoracic (chest) part of the diaphragm. Pleura lining the ribs is called costal (rib) pleura, and that which lies in the neck is the cervical (neck) pleura. Because the pleural layers are in close contact with each other, movement of the chest wall or diaphragm is transmitted to the lungs, and vice versa.

Between the two layers of pleura is a slight exudate (layer of moisture) which lubricates the surfaces, thus preventing friction between the lungs and chest wall during breathing.

Muscles of Respiration

Several muscles are involved in breathing:

- the diaphragm (see page 10)
- the intercostals (between the ribs)
- scalene muscles
- sternocleidomastoid muscles
- abdominal muscles.

Also coming into play in the breathing process are the trapezius, the parasternal (beside the breastbone) and the pectoralis muscles.

The intercostals (internal and external) connect the bony arches between the ribs. During breathing, the intercostal muscles between each pair of ribs contract (shorten), causing the ribs to swing outwards and upwards. The pairs work together with the diaphragm to draw air into the lungs.

The scalene muscles, situated deep on each side of the neck, elevate the first and second ribs during inspiration (inhalation) to enlarge the upper chest cavity and stabilize the chest wall.

The two sternocleidomastoid muscles (referring to the breastbone and collarbone) muscles arise from each side of the breastbone and inner part of the collarbone (clavicle). When breathing requires increased effort, these muscles come into play along with the scalene muscles. They elevate the breastbone during inspiration and slightly enlarge the chest cavity.

The abdominal muscles (four sets, forming a sort of 'corset') compress the lower ribs to assist in forced expiration.

The two trapezius muscles extend from the backbone (spine) and base of the skull, across the back and shoulders, to join the scapulae (shoulderblades; singular: scapula) and the clavicle. They pull the head and shoulders backwards.

The parasternal muscles are those on either side of the breastbone.

The pectoralis muscles, commonly known as the pectorals, are fan-shaped muscles situated on each side of the chest. They are attached to the collarbones, humerus (upper arm bone), breastbone, and costal cartilage (on the ribs). The pectoral muscles pull the arms towards the body and aid in chest expansion.

THE DIAPHRAGM

The diaphragm, considered the major muscle of inspiration, is a dome-shaped sheet of muscle and tendon located between the chest and abdominal cavities. Its anterior (front) surface is attached to sternal (breastbone) cartilage, the posterior (back) section is attached to the lumbar vertebrae (spinal bones at the small of the back), and the lateral (side) segments are attached to the chest wall in the area of the lower seven ribs.

Quiet breathing is accomplished primarily by the alternate contraction and relaxation of the diaphragm. When you inhale, your diaphragm contracts, or tightens, and its dome lowers. This increases the length of the chest cavity. As the diaphragm moves downwards, it compresses the abdomen. At the same time, muscles controlling the ribs contract, pulling them outwards and enlarging the chest cavity from side to side and from back to front.

With chest enlargement comes an expansion of the elastic lungs to fill the increased space. A vacuum is in effect created and air is sucked into the lungs by way of the nose, trachea, bronchi and small airway divisions. The process of inhalation thus occurs.

Diaphragmatic action has been compared with that of a piston, which moves downwards and upwards, creating pressure changes within the chest cavity, and so causing air to move in and out of the lungs.

Exhalation (breathing out) takes place when the forces that produced lung expansion are released, similar to the way a balloon shrinks back to its original size once the air is let out. Air is forced outwards by relaxation of the muscles and by the elastic recoil of the lungs. The diaphragm relaxes and resumes its dome shape, and the rib cage assumes its resting dimensions.

Fig. 6. Diaphragm during inhalation   **Fig. 7. Diaphragm during exhalation**

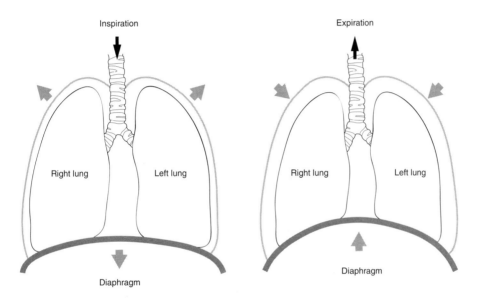

When breathing requires more effort, the external intercostal muscles and the accessory muscles (such as the scalene and sternocleidomastoid) are recruited to help.

It is interesting to note that the sac that encloses the heart (the pericardium) is attached at its base to the diaphragm and in front to the breastbone. The significance of this will become clear when you read later about the advantages of breathing diaphragmatically (see pages 115–116).

Gas Exchange

The primary function of the respiratory system is to provide oxygen for the body's metabolic needs and to remove carbon dioxide from the tissues. (Metabolism is the sum of all the chemical changes that take place within an organism.)

BREATHING AND CIRCULATION

When air is inhaled, it travels through the trachea and into the bronchi – each supplying a lung. The bronchi then branch, like limbs of a tree, finally becoming microscopic structures and ending in a series of alveoli. These resemble bubbles and have very thin walls, only one cell thick. It is here that the exchange of gases, mentioned above, takes place.

Surrounding the alveoli is a network of tiny blood vessels called capillaries. They are thin enough to allow blood cells to squeeze through them. Oxygen from inspired (inhaled) air reaches the alveoli and moves into the bloodstream by way of the capillaries that surround them, in exchange for carbon dioxide which is excreted in expired (exhaled) air.

Red blood cells contain a transport protein called hemoglobin. Hemoglobin contains iron, and this strongly attracts oxygen molecules. In the lungs, molecules of hemoglobin bind with oxygen to form a compound called oxyhemoglobin. Oxyhemoglobin carries oxygen around in the blood, releasing it wherever it is needed.

Following the exchange of gases in the alveoli, the blood suffusing the lungs is rich in oxygen and poor in carbon dioxide. It is returned to the left side of the heart, which pumps it throughout the body. As the blood flows through the body, red blood cells deliver the oxygen they contain to various tissues, picking up carbon dioxide at the same time. When the blood eventually arrives at the right side of the heart, it is oxygen-poor and carbon dioxide-rich, and ready to be pumped through the lungs again. As it passes through the lungs, oxygen from inhaled air passes into the bloodstream (via the alveoli) in exchange for carbon dioxide, which is then breathed out. The cycle thus repeats itself again and again.

Fig. 8. Blood circulation and gas exchange

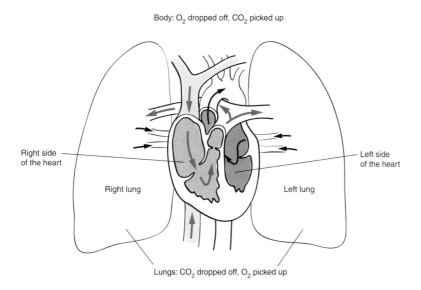

Body: O_2 dropped off, CO_2 picked up

Right side of the heart

Left side of the heart

Right lung

Left lung

Lungs: CO_2 dropped off, O_2 picked up

NERVE CONTROL

Although largely automatic and usually involuntary, the act of breathing is controlled by centers in the brain. These are actually groups of scattered neurons (nerve cells) that function as a unit. They regulate respiratory rate, depth and rhythm.

CHEMICAL CONTROL

Carbon dioxide is an acid chemical substance which stimulates the respiratory center to send out the impulses that act on the muscles involved in breathing. It is this which is the ultimate factor in controlling and regulating the frequency, rate and depth of respiration.

Both controls – nerve and chemical – are essential: without either, you could not continue to breathe on your own.

Conclusion

As you read on, you will now have an understanding of how the exercises described later in this book can help. This, I hope, will encourage you to persevere with them, and to integrate them into your daily activities. As such, they will become an eagerly anticipated and pleasurable experience, rather than something to 'get over with', or as measures to take only when encountering breathing difficulties.

First, we will take a look in Chapter 2 at asthma symptoms and triggers, and at current treatments available.

Understanding Asthma

Asthma is a common chronic disorder of the respiratory system, in which the muscular tubes through which air flows into and out of the lungs (the airways) tighten, a state referred to as broncho-constriction. The airways also become inflamed, swollen and hyper-reactive, and an excess of mucus is produced. These responses are the result of various stimuli to which the airways are exposed, mainly irritants known as 'triggers'. They cause the airways to contract, thus limiting airflow.

Asthma Symptoms

Asthma comes from a Greek word that means 'panting', and this characterizes what happens during an episode.

The bronchi and the larger bronchioles are surrounded by tiny bands of smooth muscle. When these contract in response to a trigger, the airways become narrower, so that less oxygen passes into and out of the lungs with each respiration. Breathing becomes difficult (dyspnea, also known as dyspnoea in the UK), and the person experiencing the asthma episode may assume a hunched-over posture in an attempt to obtain more air. The bronchial tubes also become irritated and inflamed, causing the bronchial walls to swell and produce excess mucus. The mucus may form plugs, and so aggravate airway obstruction.

Fig. 9. Normal small airway

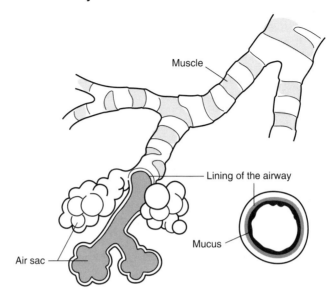

Muscle

Lining of the airway

Mucus

Air sac

Fig. 10. Small airway during asthma episode

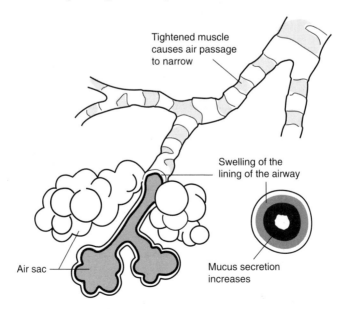

Tightened muscle
causes air passage
to narrow

Swelling of the
lining of the airway

Air sac

Mucus secretion
increases

With the resulting limited airflow into and out of the lungs, gas exchange in the alveoli becomes less effective. Body cells receive less oxygen, and carbon dioxide builds up. The urge to breathe then becomes stronger, and the person experiencing an asthma episode becomes frightened and desperate for the next breath.

Other asthma symptoms include:

- wheezing
- tightness in the chest
- retractions (sucking in of the chest or neck skin)
- coughing episodes (often preceded by laughing or crying)
- fatigue
- tingling in the fingers and toes (due to hyperventilation, or overbreathing).

Who Is Susceptible to Asthma?

Asthma can affect anyone of any nationality, but it most frequently appears in young children. It is, in fact, responsible for more absences from school and work than any other chronic illness, at great monetary cost to society.

Asthma is more common in families where at least one person has the condition. The link appears stronger if it is the mother who has asthma. These individuals are born with a tendency toward having hyper-reactive airways. Their breathing passages over-react to agents in the environment that do not affect most people.

Asthma occurs about twice as often in infants who live with a parent who smokes. Exposure to tobacco smoke also increases the risk for infants to develop allergies.

Asthma Triggers

A trigger is anything that can provoke an episode or make it worse. Asthma episodes may be precipitated by air pollution, such as that from industrial and photochemical smog outdoors, and from indoor pollutants such as those from cooking and heating sources. Smoking, either active or passive (second-hand smoke) is especially irritating to the respiratory system. Exposure of an unborn child, infant or young child to tobacco smoke increases the risk of asthma. Other triggers include:

- plant pollens
- flowers
- grass
- animal dander (small scales from the hair or feathers of birds)
- dust mites
- molds
- cockroaches
- some foods and medications
- cold air
- some forms of exercise.

Although an infectious illness may trigger an asthma episode, asthma itself is not spread by germs, and it is not contagious.

Emotional stress, although not a cause of asthma, can undoubtedly provoke episodes or aggravate them.

Allergies

Allergy (from Greek *allos,* meaning 'other', and *ergon,* 'work') describes an altered reaction of body tissues to a specific substance (allergen) which, in non-sensitive persons, will in similar amounts produce no adverse effect.

Well-known allergic conditions include asthma, ear and eye allergies, and hay fever.

Allergies play a key role in asthma, and special skin tests can be done to help to identify allergens that may be triggering the condition or causing chronic inflammation.

Diagnosing Asthma

Many of the symptoms of asthma are similar to those of other respiratory illnesses, such as emphysema and chronic bronchitis. Proper diagnosis is therefore essential, so as to give asthma sufferers the best possible chances of a long and productive life.

A competent doctor will perform a thorough investigation, which usually starts with taking notes on personal and family history. A family history of allergy could indicate asthma. Medication history is also pertinent: if you take aspirin, for example, it could be an asthma trigger.

The doctor will also wish to know when the illness started, what symptoms you've experienced, when and how severe the episodes have been, and what factors appear to make them worse. In addition, he or she will want to know what drugs you have taken to relieve your symptoms, and what effect these medicines have had. Finally, it is important to inform your doctor of any life-threatening complications that have occurred in connection with your symptoms.

After collecting relevant information, the doctor will then perform a physical examination. He or she will use a stethoscope to listen for sounds such as wheezing, although this is usually present only during an asthma episode. The next step is to check the muscles used in breathing, to determine if they appear overused – another sign of possible asthma.

Chest X-rays can confirm suspected airway obstruction, especially if they are taken when an individual is experiencing breathing difficulties. Usually, however, the lungs of a person with asthma look normal between episodes, unless there has been previous damage to them.

The doctor will also order blood tests, including a blood count. Some people with asthma have an abnormally high number of eosinophils. These are white blood cells that fight allergies and parasitic infections. They increase during the healing stage of inflammation, and are very active in the later stages.

Blood tests can also help diagnose any other disorder that may complicate asthma or its treatment.

Also helpful in diagnosing asthma is an analysis of sputum, which may reveal the presence of eosinophils and various particles such as destroyed cells and fragments of molds.

PULMONARY FUNCTION TESTS

Pulmonary (lung) function tests are usually done to determine the presence and severity of airway obstruction. One group of such tests is known as *spirometry* (from the Latin word *spirare*, 'to breathe', and the Greek word *metron*, meaning 'measure'). An instrument called a spirometer is used to measure the amount of air taken into the lungs at different points in the breathing cycle. The patient breathes into a mouthpiece connected by a tube to a machine that measure the volume of air inhaled and exhaled. The results are plotted on a graph.

Another diagnostic test for asthma is the *methacholine challenge*, which is a method of measuring airway activity. A saline aerosol is inhaled as a control, followed by increasing concentrations of a drug called methacholine chloride. This substance slightly narrows the airways and so helps determine responsiveness. The test is used to confirm a diagnosis of asthma when symptoms are present.

Exercise testing can also be done to help in diagnosing exercise-induced asthma. In the exercise test, the person suspected of having asthma is asked to ride an exercise bicycle or run on a treadmill while breathing cold air. Afterwards, he or she repeats the pulmonary-function test done prior to exercising. If the individual has asthma and his or her airways are hyper-responsive, testing should show airflow obstruction, which indicates narrowing of the airways.

This procedure is carried out under close observation and usually requires fewer than 10 minutes of exercise.

ALLERGY TESTING

Since allergies are among the most common asthma triggers, allergy testing is an important diagnostic tool.

Evidence of allergy may be obtained through blood tests that detect the presence of specific antibodies to various allergens. (An antibody, also known as immunoglobulin, or Ig, is a specific substance produced by a person or animal in response to the presence of an antigen.) An increased number of eosinophils is often associated with allergies. An elevated level of IgE antibodies also suggests allergies. (The IgE antibody is one of five classes of antibody. It is implicated in allergic reactions such as hay fever, hives and asthma.)

One such testing technique is known as RAST (Radio-Allergo-Sorbent Test). This method is considered less accurate than skin testing (see below), although it may be useful for certain individuals. It is more expensive compared with skin testing, and it takes longer to obtain results.

Faster and less expensive than the RAST is a relatively new technique called MAST (Multiple Antigen Simultaneous Testing). This has been developed for measuring allergen-specific IgE antibodies. It provides accurate results which are usually available within a week.

Additional evaluation may include allergy skin testing for specific allergens that may trigger asthma episodes. In use for over 100 years, this method is very reliable in determining the presence of allergy to a specific substance. It is performed by pricking, scratching or injecting the skin with a small amount of the suspected allergen. A positive reaction is judged by the amount of swelling that occurs in 20–30 minutes. Skin testing is time-consuming, however, and in highly sensitive individuals may produce all-over body reactions.

PEAK FLOW METER

One procedure that people with asthma can do at home involves a hand-held device called a peak flow meter. It is a popular tool, and a useful one for those who are able to monitor their own asthma. It measures the speed at which air flows from the lungs during the first 150 milliseconds of rapid exhalation. When the reading indicates a decrease in air flow, it may be a sign of bronchospasm (spasm of the bronchus), which signals that an asthma episode may be developing.

Some doctors suggest the routine use of a peak flow meter, to be used first thing in the morning and again just before going to bed for the night. Monitoring with this device can alert an asthma sufferer to an imminent episode, and so enable him or her to institute treatment as early as possible.

RATING SEVERITY

Rating the severity of a patient's asthma symptoms helps the doctor devise the most effective individual treatment plan possible. Asthma specialists now distinguish four categories of severity based on the frequency of symptoms or episodes, and results of pulmonary function tests:

1. mild intermittent, when random episodes occur less than twice a week, and night-time symptoms occur less than once a month
2. mild persistent, when daytime symptoms occur more than twice a week but less than once a day, and night-time symptoms occur more than twice a month
3. moderate persistent, when some symptoms occur every day, and night-time symptoms occur more than once a week

4. severe persistent, when daytime symptoms are continual and night-time symptoms are frequent.

Preventive Measures

Avoiding asthma triggers is the best form of prevention. Of the many allergens implicated in asthma episodes, house dust is perhaps the most difficult to eradicate. Dust-collectors abound in many homes, especially in children's rooms. These include carpets, curtains, bookshelves, stuffed toys, pillows, mattresses and bedclothes.

Here is a brief list of broad types of allergens and suggested preventive measures:

Allergen	Preventive Measure
Indoor allergens	Try as far as possible to keep the home dust-free, by: eliminating carpets, curtains and other dust-collectors; using mattress/pillow covers; improving ventilation and decreasing humidity; cleaning regularly
Tobacco smoke	Limit or eliminate exposure to passive (second-hand) smoke
Outdoor pollutants	Decrease level of motor vehicle emissions Decrease airborne commercial and industrial pollutants
Workplace allergens	Prevent exposure of workers to harmful workplace agents Prevent sensitization by adequate occupational hygiene measures
Respiratory infections	Prevent respiratory infections among young children by: promoting good nutrition; avoiding overcrowded daycare centers; making sure daycare/nursery settings maintain infection-control measures

Food Allergies · Breastfeeding for at least the first six months has been shown to reduce significantly the likelihood that a child will develop food allergies later in life

Treating Asthma

The key to treating asthma successfully is self-management. This is not to say that people with asthma should dispense with the services of a doctor and rely entirely on themselves for managing their condition. *It is imperative that you work in close collaboration with a qualified, competent health care professional, and follow faithfully any plan he or she devises for you.* Along with your doctor's guidance, however, you can use the natural resources you have with and within you (your body, your mind and your breath) to recapture a measure of control over your life, enjoy the confidence resulting therefrom, and experience an enhanced sense of well-being and productivity.

THE DOCTOR-PATIENT PARTNERSHIP

Doctors will tell you that patient involvement is crucial to the successful management of chronic disorders such as asthma. As a patient (or friend or relative of someone with asthma), the data which you provide the doctor is vital. The concerns you express and the pertinent information you give will help the doctor develop the most effective individualized treatment plan for managing or eliminating asthma symptoms.

ASTHMA JOURNAL

An asthma journal/diary can be an important self-management tool. With the help of a diary, you can monitor your condition and make careful notes of things such as:

- when episodes occur
- what you were doing when they took place
- when episodes tend to occur (in the morning, at night, following vigorous exercise, or in certain kinds of weather, for example)
- your symptoms.

Keeping a record of this kind will help you form a clearer picture of your condition, and could assist your doctor in creating the most effective treatment plan. Any information relating to your condition will make managing your asthma easier, and increase the likelihood of the best possible outcome.

Once you have gained a sense of being an active, contributing participant in your own health, you will be more likely to stick to any treatment program and therefore improve your chances of achieving control over your asthma.

ASTHMA MEDICATION

Caution: If you have asthma, it is imperative that you use only those medicines prescribed for you by your doctor. Self-medication with over-the-counter (OTC) drugs could prove deadly. Do not use any herbal preparation or dietary supplement without first consulting your doctor or other qualified therapist.

There's a wide range of medications used to treat asthma. Those in current use, however, fall into two broad categories: quick-relief medicines and controller medicines.

Quick-relief Medicines

These are used to treat asthma episodes. They include a class of drugs known as beta-agonists, such as salbutamol (albuterol). They relax the smooth muscles that tighten around airways and limit airflow to the lungs. These medicines are also called bronchodilators, since they widen the air passages and so improve airflow.

Included in this category is ipratropium bromide, which also opens airways during an asthma episode, though not as rapidly and completely as the beta-agonists.

Controller Medicines

These are used to prevent and reduce airway inflammation. The most effective are inhaled steroids. They reduce existing inflammation and also help to prevent its recurrence. Beclomethasone is an example of this type of medicine.

Also in this category are cromolyn and nedocromil. These do not reduce inflammation that is already present, but do prevent it from developing.

These medicines are usually taken daily by metered-dose inhaler (MDI).

Other controller medicines include long-acting beta-agonists such as salmeterol (Serevent), which is administered by inhaler, the short-acting salbutamol (albuterol), which is taken by mouth (orally), and leukotriene modifiers such as zafirlukast and theophylline.

In addition, oral steroids such as prednisone and prednisolone may be prescribed for use every day or every other day as long-term treatments of severe persistent asthma.

Side-effects

Adverse reactions to asthma medication in long-standing use, such as salbutamol (albuterol) are not, as a rule, a serious medical concern. If, however, you are worried about any symptoms you believe to be related to your medication, be sure to discuss this with your doctor.

Inhaled steroids, though very effective as controller medicines for asthma, can produce symptoms such as hoarseness and yeast infection of the mouth (moniliasis). These medicines have also been associated, in older asthma sufferers, with an increased risk of cataracts (opacity of the lens of the eye, or its capsule, or both), glaucoma (a disease of the eye characterized by an increase in pressure inside the eyeball) and osteoporosis (increased porousness and associated brittleness of the bones). In children, these drugs have been linked with an increased risk of reduced growth (in height).

Oral steroids, despite their effectiveness, can produce adverse reactions if taken for more than 14 days a year. This, however, is rarely necessary.

A few medicines, including beta-blockers (which block the action of beta-agonist agents and responses of the sympathetic nervous system) can worsen asthma.

Reducing Side-effects
You can reduce certain undesired effects of some of the asthma medications by, for example, using a holding chamber to administer inhaled medicines, and rinsing your mouth out after each dose. (A holding chamber is a device used with a metered dose inhaler that holds the medicine mist so as to enhance its effect.)

Generally, inhaled medicines are less likely to produce adverse effects than those taken orally or injected. This is because the medication is deposited in the airways and lungs, with only a small amount absorbed by the blood.

MEDICATION GUIDELINES

Here are some guidelines for the safe and effective use of asthma medications:

* Use reminders about when to take your medicine, such as a note on the bathroom mirror, an alarm clock or by enlisting the help of a family member or friend.
* Keep to a regular schedule, taking your medicine at about the same time every day.
* Carry your inhaler with you at all times. Keep a spare inhaler at home, and perhaps also at work.
* Do not alter the dosage of any medications your doctor has prescribed for you.

- If you experience any unpleasant symptoms you believe are caused by your medicine (such as shakiness, hoarseness, headaches, irregular heartbeats) or anything that causes you concern, do not hesitate to discuss them with your doctor.
- Be sure to ask your doctor everything you need to know about your medicines. Make sure you understand explanations and directions. Ask to be shown how to use your inhaler correctly.
- Be sure to consult your doctor before using any OTC (over-the-counter) drugs. Some medicines interact, making one or both (or all of them) less effective. Two different medicines taken simultaneously may also increase their potency or produce more pronounced unwanted side-effects.
- Keep all medicines out of children's reach.
- Store medicines away from heat and direct sunlight.
- Note the expiry dates on medications, and safely discard any outdated ones.

Asthma in Pregnancy

It is estimated that asthma complicates 4–6 per cent of all pregnancies. In about one-third of women asthma sufferers, asthma improves during pregnancy; in one-third it remains the same as in pre-pregnancy, and in one-third it becomes worse.

Women with asthma, however, should not be afraid to become pregnant. With close monitoring and careful control before and during pregnancy, there should be no problems carrying a child or giving birth.

POSSIBLE COMPLICATIONS

Studies have shown that pregnant women with asthma that is not being controlled properly tend to experience complications. These include premature birth, low birthweight babies, and even perinatal mortality (death of the fetus or infant between the 28th week of pregnancy and 28th day following the birth). Pregnant women with severe asthma may develop hypertension (high blood pressure), toxemia (blood poisoning) or a complicated labor.

Some women may be afraid that taking asthma medication during pregnancy could harm their baby. Taking asthma medicines prescribed by your doctor is, however, much less likely to harm the baby than living with asthma that is poorly or ineffectively controlled. As always, do discuss with your doctor any medicines you are taking or plan to take during pregnancy.

TREATING ASTHMA IN PREGNANCY

The treatment of asthma during pregnancy varies little from that for other sufferers. The principle underlying managing the condition at this time is that the developing fetus depends on maternal circulation for its oxygen supply. If the mother's asthma is poorly controlled, her oxygen levels may be depleted, with consequent threat to the baby's development. Medicines for treating asthma are, therefore, usually maintained, though any judged unsafe will be withdrawn.

Pregnancy can exacerbate conditions such as rhinitis (inflammation of nasal mucous membranes) and sinusitis (inflammation of the sinuses). In fact, sinusitis is about six times more prevalent in pregnant women. To help in reducing these conditions, nasal washing with saline (salt water) is recommended (see page 125).

Labor and Delivery
It is particularly important, for both mother and baby, to maintain an adequate oxygen supply during labor and delivery. Regularly scheduled asthma medications will, therefore, usually be continued throughout labor.

After Delivery
Although asthma medicines are commonly found in breastmilk tested for their presence, this should not deter mothers with asthma from breastfeeding. Inhaled medicines such as the beta-agonists, inhaled steroids, and cromolyn have not been

found in significant levels in breastmilk to produce ill-effects in an infant. Please be certain to consult your doctor if you have any concerns in this matter.

CONTROL GUIDELINES

You can do a lot to achieve and maintain the best possible control of your asthma symptoms during pregnancy:

- Reduce your exposure to asthma triggers, especially tobacco smoke.
- Take all prescribed medicines faithfully.
- Consult your doctor about measures to take against possible viral infections.
- Exercise moderately according to a regimen approved by your doctor, with proper precautions.
- Help your obstetrician manage your asthma by informing him or her of all medicines you are using, and of any breathing difficulties you may experience.

Asthma in Childhood

Parents need to be well informed about the nature of asthma, its signs and symptoms, preventive measures and prescribed treatments. This information should also be shared with other family members, baby-sitters, teachers, the school nurse and anyone else involved in their child's daily routine.

Taking good care of a child with asthma, and managing his or her condition competently, may at first seem daunting. Being equipped with the right information, however, will help you develop the necessary skills.

Be on the alert for the four main signs of asthma: coughing, wheezing, retractions (see pages 15-17) and quickened breathing. Regularly assess the child's condition and follow meticulously the proper medication schedule prescribed by your doctor. With time and practice, parents and other care-givers will become confident in providing the best possible care for the child with asthma.

On page xv there is a list of yoga postures and breathing exercises that are appropriate and helpful for children. These can be incorporated into the child's treatment plan.

VISITS TO THE DOCTOR

When assessing a child's asthma status, doctors rely more on the patient's medical history and physical findings than on pulmonary (lung) function measurements. This is particularly true of children under the age of five, because of their inability to use a peak flow meter accurately, for example.

For children in this age group, some doctors suggest that two adults be present during a visit: one to look after the child, and one to pay rapt attention to what the doctor says, as this could include:

- important information about the four signs of asthma, and how to score them
- how to use a holding chamber
- how to arrive at the best possible treatment plan

ASTHMA IN INFANCY

Infants with asthma present special challenges to parents and doctors because problems tend to develop fairly rapidly. The airways of children under 12 months of age are much smaller than those of older children, and can become blocked more easily. An infant's condition can therefore deteriorate much more quickly during an episode.

Moreover, infants cannot, of course, tell their parents that their chest feels tight or that they are having difficulty breathing. In addition, new parents with little experience may not have learned how to judge the severity of an asthma episode.

Viral infections, such as viral bronchitis or pneumonia, are the most common cause of asthma in children of six months of age or younger. Signs of asthma in this age group include:

- a change in the child's cry
- an inability to suckle or feed
- an increased breathing rate
- a change in skin color.

CONTROL GUIDELINES

- To reduce the chances of your child developing allergies (which can lead to asthma), do try to breastfeed for at least the first four to six months. Also, consult with your doctor or a qualified nutritionist when it comes time to wean your baby onto solid foods.
- Minimize your child's exposure, as far as possible, to allergens and irritants, especially tobacco smoke. Also, try to keep pets out of the home – and choose a baby-sitter who does the same.
- Keep the child's bedroom as dust-free and clean as possible. Wash bedding often in hot water; use allergy-free mattress covers and pillow cases; avoid using carpeting, curtains and other havens for dust mites and mold spores.
- Maintain as normal a routine as possible for your child, with minimal or no restrictions on activities, including exercise. This will do much to reinforce a positive attitude in the child toward his or her condition, and help to build up his or her self-esteem and confidence.
- Use appropriate yoga postures and breathing techniques (see page xv) to help control and alleviate the child's symptoms and asthma episodes.
- The school nurse and the child's teachers should be made aware of the child's condition, and have a record of your doctor's name, telephone number and a list of medications in current use.

Conclusion

Asthma has now reached almost epidemic proportions in several of the world's industrialized nations. Many people who know they have the disorder, however, do not appreciate that with available treatment they can lead active lives that include being able to exercise and participate in sports. Indeed, many high-achieving athletes have asthma.

The range of treatment options for asthma is wide, and includes education, environmental control measures, anti-asthma medicines, and a number of respected adjunct therapies. Individualized treatment and control strategies should be discussed with your doctor, and you should consider yourself an invaluable component of the doctor–patient partnership.

Perhaps the most important aspect of asthma management is education. It is futile to treat a person experiencing an asthma episode with 'wonder' drugs and then send him or her back to the same environment that contributed to the episode in the first place. He or she must be given the right information to deal with offending environmental pollutants.

Many clinics and doctors' offices have educational literature for patients and their relatives/carers. Some have nurse-educators who will review and discuss treatments and any other areas of concern, and who can demonstrate the correct way to use an MDI ('puffer'), both with and without a spacer device. Many organizations devoted to respiratory health (see Resource Organizations chapter) have websites that provide useful information on asthma. Do avail yourself of these wonderful resources. Remember: the better informed you are about asthma, the more effectively you can help manage it, and the better will be your quality of life.

The Yoga Approach

Yoga is fast becoming one of the most sought-after exercise and training methods. It is the basis of many stress-reduction and health-promotion programs, as well as of many childbirth preparation classes. It is also used as adjunctive therapy for a number of health disorders, including respiratory ailments such as asthma. In fact, there are now many breathing rehabilitation clinics that teach clients certain techniques based on the yogic voluntary controlled breathing practices known collectively as *pranayama*.

What Is Yoga?

A system of physical and mental training for fitness and personal development, yoga is based on sound anatomical and physiological principles. Its origins can be traced to the Indian subcontinent 4,000 years ago, and it has withstood the test of time. It is an approach to wellness that promotes the harmonious working-together of the human being's three components: body, mind, and spirit. It should be noted, however, that although yoga developed alongside Hinduism and other religions, it has never been considered a religious practice. It can therefore be practiced with complete confidence by anyone, regardless of his or her beliefs.

There are different kinds of yoga, but the one most readily embraced by the millions of people worldwide who are practicing it today is Hatha Yoga.

Hatha Yoga consists of:

- Non-strenuous stretching and strengthening exercises (*asanas*), which take each joint in the body through its full range of motion. The exercises are done with awareness, in synchronization with regular breathing. They benefit not only joints and muscles, but also other bodily structures such as organs and glands.
- Exercises in voluntary controlled respiration, collectively known as *pranayama*. They train you in the most efficient way of breathing; one that requires a minimum of effort in return for a maximum intake of oxygen. They also provide a 'tool' for helping you cope with difficult emotions.
- Concentration, meditation and relaxation techniques, which help to divert attention from disturbing environmental stimuli and so train you to become calmer and more focused. This leads to a sense of greater personal control and empowerment, and a feeling of not being totally at the mercy of outside influences (an attribute of immense value to those experiencing the anxiety which can accompany an asthma episode). Practicing these exercises regularly is also useful in helping you to counteract fatigue, which is often a concomitant of asthma.

The yoga approach to attaining and maintaining optimum health also includes attention to good hygiene and adequate nutrition. Yoga is not, however, a quick fix. The benefits you derive from its practice will be proportionate to the time and perseverance you give to it.

BENEFITS

Physical benefits of the regular practice of yoga include:

- improved efficiency of the lungs and cardiovascular system
- less oxygen requirement for muscles
- more efficient use of respiratory muscles (see page 9)
- less likelihood of breathing difficulties, such as shortness of breath and hyperventilation (see pages 143–144)

- improved posture
- improved flexibility; better range of motion of joints
- reduced muscle tension; less fatigue
- reduced likelihood of being overweight.

Psychological benefits of regular yoga practice can include:

- an enhanced sense of well-being
- increased self-confidence
- greater self-esteem
- the ability to relax more easily
- better quality sleep
- improved concentration
- reduced chances of anxiety, panic and depression
- fewer cravings for tobacco, food and alcohol.

Guidelines for Safe Practice

Before starting this or any other exercise program, please check with your doctor and obtain his or her permission.

GENERAL CAUTIONS

Pregnant women who have a history of actual or threatened miscarriage are cautioned not to do the exercises in the first three or four months of pregnancy. If the pregnancy is progressing normally, you may try the warm-ups in Chapter 4, omitting the Lying Twist and the Sun Salutations. But first check with your doctor.

Not recommended for practice during pregnancy are the lying postures in the prone (face-downwards) position, such as the Cobra, the Half

Locust and the Bow. Avoid lying flat on your back after the first trimester (three months) to prevent restriction of the blood and oxygen flow to mother and fetus, through pressure on the inferior vena cava (principal vein draining the lower part of the body).

If you suffer from an ear or eye condition or have an eye disorder such as a detached retina, omit the inverted postures such as the Half and Full Shoulderstand (pages 99–101). If you suffer from epilepsy, avoid the Cat Stretch postures (pages 53–54).

Avoid inverted postures and rapid abdominal breathing if you have high blood pressure. If you have heart disease, avoid inverted postures, the Half Locust (page 84) and the Bow (pages 85–87).

Omit practice of the inverted postures during the monthly menstrual period.

If you have a hernia, avoid the Camel posture (page 91), the Cobra (page 88), the Half Locust (page 84) and the Bow (page 85).

Avoid the Fish (page 83) and the Camel (page 91) if you have a thyroid gland problem or neck pain.

If you have varicose veins, omit the Sun Salutations (pages 55–59). If you have venous blood clots, avoid sitting for any length of time in the folded-legs postures, such as the Perfect Posture (page 63).

Preparation

Before engaging in any exercise it is imperative that you warm up your body. Please spend 5 to 10 minutes doing so. Do not exercise within two hours of eating a heavy meal. This caution is particularly important if you have a history of angina (severe pain and constriction about the heart).

When to Practice

Try to do the exercises at about the same time every day (or at least every other day) on a regular basis.

Practicing in the morning helps reduce stiffness after many hours spent in bed, and gives you energy for your day. Practicing in the evening produces a pleasant tiredness and promotes sound sleep. If you find, however, that evening practice is too stimulating and prevents you from falling asleep easily, then try instead to fit your exercises in where they seem most convenient and beneficial.

If you plan a session of breathing exercises (*pranayama*) separate from the physical exercises (*asanas*), make it about 15 minutes after doing the simpler *asanas*, or about an hour before. You may also plan two 15-minute or half-hour sessions a day, or every other day: warm-ups and other exercises in the morning, and breathing and meditative exercises in the evening.

FITTING YOGA INTO YOUR DAY

Several of the exercises, such as the neck and shoulder warm-ups (see pages 47–48) and also some of the breathing techniques in Chapter 5, can be done at convenient times throughout the day, to prevent a buildup of tension. For example, you can tighten your abdominal muscles as you exhale while sitting at a desk or standing in line. You can slow down your breathing and make it smoother and deeper when you feel stressed, such as while driving in difficult traffic conditions, to help you stay calm.

Where to Practice

Choose a quiet, well-ventilated room with soft lighting. Because concentration is crucial to the effectiveness of yoga practice, arrange to be undisturbed for the expected duration of your exercise session.

Practice on an even surface, and if the room is not carpeted, place a non-skid mat on the floor on which to do your exercises. When it is warm enough, practice outdoors, on a patio or lawn on which a mat is spread.

From now on, I shall refer to the surface on which you practice as the 'mat'.

Comfort and Hygiene

Remove from your person any object that might injure you, such as glasses, hair ornaments or jewellery. Wear loose, comfortable clothing that permits you to move and breathe freely. Practice barefoot whenever possible.

For maximum comfort, empty your bladder, and possibly also your bowel, before starting yoga practice. If you wish, you may have a warm (not hot) bath or shower before exercising, especially if you feel particularly stiff. Attend as well to oral and nasal hygiene (see pages 125–126).

Food and Drink

Practicing with a full stomach impedes the free movement of your diaphragm. Yoga exercises are best practiced on an empty or near-empty stomach. The best time for practice is before breakfast. At this time, however, after 8 to 10 or so hours in bed without food, your blood sugar will be low – it is preferable to drink a glass of juice and eat something light, rather than exercise on a completely empty stomach.

Generally, however, it is advisable to allow two or three hours to elapse after a meal, depending on its size and content, before practicing. You may practice an hour after eating a light snack. If you find this difficult or inconvenient, you may drink a cup of tea or other non-alcoholic beverage prior to exercising.

Setting the Scene

With some forms of exercise, it is not unusual to be 'working out' while thinking of unrelated matters: what you are going to cook for dinner tomorrow; what you are going to wear to school or work; how well you are going to do in a test or interview, or how you are going to meet a deadline. This is not encouraged in yoga. Without the appropriate mental setting, yoga exercises will have no lasting value. For the restoration and maintenance of good health, you need to approach yoga practice with an attitude of calm and positive anticipation.

When you arrive at the place where you are going to practice, leave behind you any cares or concerns; any grudges, resentments or other negative feelings. Before starting the exercises, spend a minute or two sitting still, with eyes closed, in quiet contemplation. You might, for example, reflect on one or two things for which to be thankful. You might simply turn your attention to your breathing and, if it is rapid and shallow, consciously slow it down by taking several deep breaths (without straining), in smooth succession. You might do a quick mental check of your body, from head to toe, and willfully let go of any tightness you detect in your jaw, hands, shoulders or elsewhere. You might, alternatively, silently recite some inspirational saying, such as: 'I will stay calm and in control,' or 'I will leave disorder behind me.' The general aim is to quiet your body and divert your mind from its usual concerns, in preparation for the yoga program ahead.

How to Practice

One characteristic of popular exercise programs of the past, and even of some current ones, was the ever-increasing number of times exercises were repeated, and the decrease in the resting period between them. Relaxation, which is a significant component of muscle activity, was thus neglected. Multiple repetitions of an exercise tend to produce fatigue and stiffness. Instead of tiresome repetitions, therefore, with this yoga program you can come back to a specific exercise later, or try a more advanced variation of it, or experiment with different combinations so as to exercise all muscle groups. Alternatively, you can give extra attention to areas of your body that need additional stretching and strengthening.

Rest periods and breathing appropriately are as important as the postures (*asanas*) themselves. Doing the exercises slowly and with complete awareness ensures control of your position and movement at all times, and helps to prevent injury. These principles are inherent in the yogic approach to exercise, one that represents centuries of wisdom.

Counter-postures

As a general rule, a backwards-bending posture should be balanced by a forwards-bending one, and vice versa. For example, after practicing the Cobra (page 88), you could do the Curling Leaf (page 78). Pregnant women could do the Single Knee Press (page 80) following the Bridge (page 81).

Warming Up

Always begin by warming up (see Chapter 4), and give full attention to what you are doing. This has already been mentioned, but it is worth repeating since it is one of the things that make yoga techniques so effective in the maintenance and restoration of good health.

Visualization

Visualize the completed posture. This is your goal, but not necessarily one that you must reach today. What really matters is your *attempt* to reach it, and the diligence and perseverance you bring to your practice. Try also to visualize the structures underneath the parts being exercised: for example, the organs, glands or blood and lymph vessels inside your body. Imagine them receiving an improved blood supply, and their waste products being thoroughly eliminated. Use any other imagery with which you are comfortable, to enhance the effects of your exercise. Be creative.

Breathing

Breathe regularly through your nostrils while doing an exercise (unless otherwise instructed). Do not hold your breath. Synchronize your breathing with the movement being executed. This allows delivery of oxygen to the working muscles, and helps to eliminate substances that cause fatigue. It also counteracts tension buildup.

Repetition and Rest

Except when doing warm-ups – in which several repetitions of an exercise in smooth succession are usual practice – do each exercise once or twice only (you can repeat it later), making your movements slow and conscious. During the holding period (indicated in the exercise instructions as 'hold'), do not simultaneously hold your breath; keep it flowing.

Always rest briefly after each exercise, and check that you are breathing regularly.

After Exercising

A period of cooling down after exercising is imperative (see Chapter 4). In addition, most yoga classes end with a top-to-toe relaxation exercise, usually the Pose of Tranquility (see page 154).

Try not to eat for at least half an hour after exercising. You may take a bath or shower after about 15 minutes.

Asthma and Exercise

Exercise can trigger an asthma episode, but it is an activity you should not avoid. If your asthma is being properly managed and it is well controlled, and if you take appropriate preventive measures, you should be able to exercise and participate in sports without experiencing bothersome symptoms.

BENEFITS FOR PEOPLE WITH ASTHMA

The benefits people with asthma can derive from exercising regularly include:

- Keeping the heart and breathing muscles strong and efficient, so that less energy is required to cope with asthma symptoms.
- Maintaining a fit and flexible body; avoiding excess weight, which can complicate asthma.
- Promoting a sense of calm, and acquiring a level of body awareness that enables you to work with your breath and use it to advantage. These benefits are particularly apparent in forms of exercise such as yoga, which involve deep breathing, mental relaxation, and meditative practices.

EXERCISE PRECAUTIONS FOR PEOPLE WITH ASTHMA

- Check with your doctor before you start any new exercise program or accelerate your progress in any you are currently practicing.
- Take your prescribed medicine before you begin to exercise, to help prevent the occurrence of asthma symptoms. Allow 15 to 30 minutes for broncho-dilators to activate in your body before you start.

The Yoga
Approach

- Use your broncho-dilator at the first sign of asthma symptoms.
- Try to exercise daily so as to maintain your strength and increase your endurance.
- Do not engage in your usual exercise when you feel ill or exhausted.
- Warm up for 5 to 15 minutes, depending on the strenuousness of your exercise program. Cool down properly afterwards. These measures alleviate drastic temperature changes in the lungs, which can trigger broncho-constriction and produce asthma symptoms.
- Avoid using perfumes, scented lotions or brightly colored items of clothing that may attract insects.
- Consider drinking small amounts of water during exercise, to keep your airways hydrated, and so prevent mucus plugs from forming and airway muscles from tightening.
- Try to breathe through your nose, as slowly as possible, to filter, warm, and moisturize the air before it reaches the lungs.
- Indoors is perhaps the safest place to exercise because the air tends to be warmer and more humid than it is outdoors. Indoor exercise also gives some protection from certain forms of pollution, such as ozone and sulfur dioxide.
- Less stressful than running, soccer, basketball, tennis and skiing are walking, golf, baseball and bicycling slowly.
- Indoor water sports offer wonderful benefits. They involve the whole body, and the warm, humid environment helps to limit the drying of the airways.
- Consult with your doctor before attempting to scuba dive, which can cause a potentially fatal injury known as barotrauma.
- When engaged in outdoor activities in cold weather, wear a mask or scarf over your face. Cold, dry air can precipitate an asthma episode.
- Do take advantage of exercise opportunities, and don't let the fear of exercise-induced asthma prevent you from leading an active, productive life. Remember to check first with your doctor.

Physical Exercises
(Asanas)

Yoga exercises are called *asanas*. An asana is a posture which is comfortably held or maintained. They are practiced slowly and mindfully, with attention fully focused on what is being done. This prevents or reduces the likelihood of inadvertent injury. They are also performed in synchronization with slow, regular breathing, usually through the nose. The completed posture is then maintained (held) for a period of time, according to individual comfort, while regular breathing continues, to provide oxygen to the working muscles. The posture is then slowly released and the starting position resumed. This is followed by a rest (recovery) period, which is a significant component of muscle activity, to prevent stiffness and a buildup of fatigue.

Warm-ups

Warm-ups are essential preparation for yoga postures. They are also imperative for people with asthma who engage in regular exercise (see page 44). They help reduce stiffness, slightly increase body temperature, and improve circulation. They are therefore useful in preventing the straining of muscles and joints once you begin practice of the exercises themselves. They help to avert the occurrence of asthma symptoms.

The warm-ups that follow have been carefully chosen because they can be integrated into activities of daily living to prevent a buildup of tension in skeletal (pertaining to the body's bony framework) muscles, and in those muscles involved in breathing.

Please do all the exercises slowly and with awareness, and do not hold your breath at any time.

The Neck

Figure-Eight
This exercise reduces stiffness and promotes flexibility in the cervical (neck) part of the spine. It also contributes to the health of respiratory structures within the neck (such as the trachea).

1   Sit comfortably. Close your eyes or keep them open. Keep your shoulders, arms, and hands relaxed. Relax your jaw and breathe regularly throughout the exercise.
2   Imagine a large figure-eight lying on its side in front of you. Starting at the middle, trace its outline with your nose, mouth or face a few times in one direction.
3   Pause briefly, then trace the outline of the imaginary figure-eight a few times in the other direction. Rest.

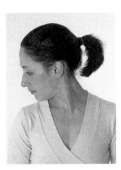

**Fig. 11.
Figure-Eight:
Head to right
chin down**

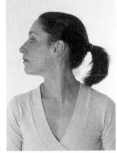

**Fig. 12.
Figure-Eight:
Head to right
chin up**

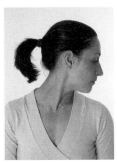

**Fig. 13.
Figure-Eight:
Head to left
chin down**

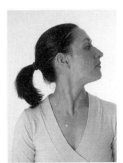

**Fig. 14.
Figure-Eight:
Head to left
chin up**

Physical Exercises

(Asanas)

Shoulder Rotation

Rotating the shoulders enhances the effects of the neck exercises. It prevents a buildup of tension in the upper back and reduces stiffness in the shoulder joints. It also improves circulation in these areas.

1   Sit comfortably. (You can also practice this exercise standing.) Observe good posture. Keep your jaw, arms, and hands relaxed. Close your eyes or keep them open. Breathe regularly throughout the exercise.
2   Lift your shoulders towards your ears to begin the rotation of the shoulders (Figure 15).
3   Bring the shoulders backwards and downwards, squeezing the shoulderblades together, and around to the front to complete one rotation (Figure 16).
4   Do a few more shoulder rotations slowly, smoothly, and with awareness.
5   Repeat the rotations in the opposite direction. Rest.

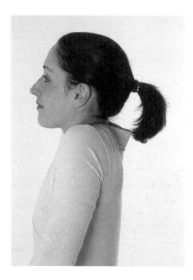

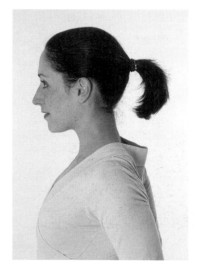

Fig. 15.
Shoulder Rotation:
Shoulders lifted towards ears

Fig. 16.
Shoulder Rotation:
Shoulders pulled backwards
and downwards

The Butterfly

The Butterfly reduces stiffness in the ankle, knee, and hip joints. It stretches and tones the muscles of the inner thighs, and also improves circulation in the lower pelvic area.

1   Sit comfortably. Hold yourself naturally erect. Relax your jaw and breathe regularly throughout the exercise.
2   Fold your legs inwards, one at a time, bringing the soles of your feet together. Clasp your hands around your feet and bring them comfortably close to your body (Figure 17).
3   Lower and raise your knees, like a butterfly flapping its wings. Do this as many times as you wish, in smooth succession (Figure 18).
4   Carefully unfold your legs and stretch them out, one at a time. Rest.

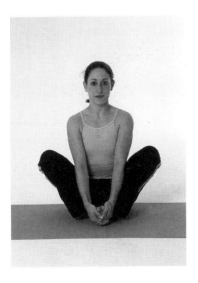

Fig. 17.
Butterfly:
Feet together, knees up

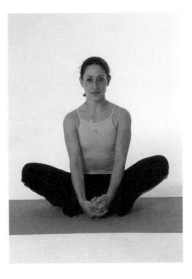

Fig. 18.
Butterfly:
Feet together, knees down

Variation: The Butterfly

1   Sit comfortably. Rest your hands on the mat behind you, with your fingers pointing backwards. Fold your legs inwards and bring the soles of your feet together (Figure 19).

2   Alternately lower and raise your knees, as many times as you wish, in smooth succession.

3   Stretch out your legs and rest.

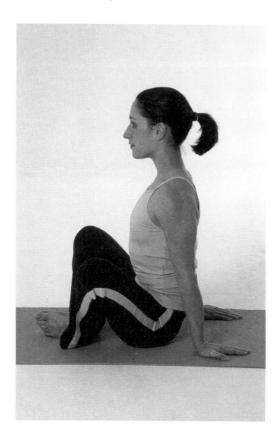

Fig. 19.
Butterfly variation:
Hands on mat

Lying Twist

This warm-up firms and strengthens the oblique and transverse abdominal muscles (part of the 'abdominal corset', see pages 9 and 68) and those of the lower back. It helps keep the midriff trim, to facilitate unrestricted movement of the diaphragm, and it promotes the health of pelvic structures.

1   Lie on your back with your arms stretched out at shoulder level. Breathe regularly.
2   Bend your legs, one at a time, and rest the soles of your feet on the mat. Now bring your knees towards your chest.
3   Keeping your shoulders and arms in firm contact with the mat, slowly, smoothly and carefully tilt your knees to one side as you exhale (Figure 20). You may keep your head still or turned to the side opposite your knees.
4   Inhale and bring your knees back to the center.
5   Exhale and tilt your knees to the opposite side, keeping your head still or turning it opposite to your knees.
6   Repeat the side-to-side tilting of your knees several times in slow, smooth succession.
7   Stretch out and rest.

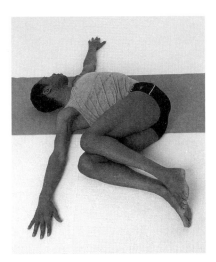

Fig. 20.
Lying Twist

Variation: Lying Twist

1   From a comfortable sitting position, lean back on your elbows.
2   Bring your knees towards your chest.
3   Alternately tilt your knees towards the left and right, in synchronization with regular breathing (Figure 21).
4   Stretch out and rest.

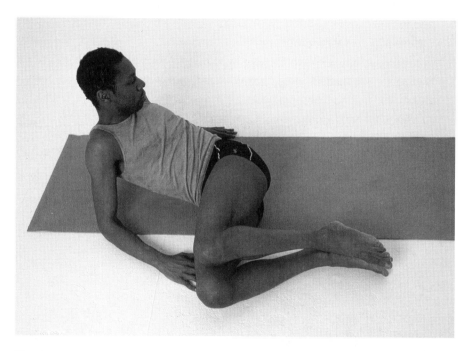

Fig. 21.
Lying Twist variation

Cat Stretch

The Cat Stretch exercises help keep your spine strong and flexible, and they are useful in preventing backache. They facilitate unrestricted breathing by reducing tension buildup in the chest and abdomen, and they improve circulation to every part of the body.

1   Get on your hands and knees, on all fours like a cat (Figure 22).
2   Exhaling, lower your head, arch your shoulders and tuck your hips down so that your entire back is rounded (Figure 23).
3   Inhale and very slowly stretch the front of your body: lift your head high and feel the front of your neck stretch gently. Stretch one leg backwards as far as you can without straining (Figure 24).
4   Exhale and lower your head. Bend the knee of your outstretched leg and bring it in towards your forehead. Feel your back muscles stretching (Figure 25).
5   Inhale and come back to your starting position (Figure 22).
6   Repeat steps 2 to 5, this time stretching out the other leg (as in step 3, Figure 24) and bringing the knee to the forehead (as in step 4, Figure 25). The two sets of exercises make one 'round'.
7   Repeat the entire exercise (round) at least once.
8   Sit or lie down and rest.

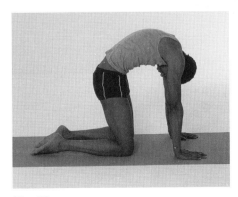

Fig. 22.
Cat Stretch:
Starting position

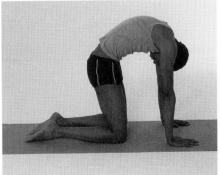

Fig. 23.
Cat Stretch:
Arched back

Physical Exercises

(Asanas)

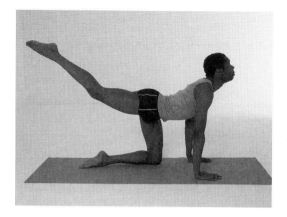

Fig. 24.
Cat Stretch:
Leg stretch

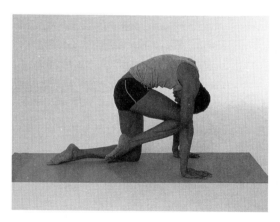

Fig. 25.
Cat Stretch:
Knee to forehead

Sun Salutations

CAUTION: Avoid these exercises if you have varicose veins, venous blood clots, high blood pressure or a hernia. See also cautions for the Dog Stretch (page 97).

In addition to being good warm-up and cool-down exercises, the Sun Salutations can be used as a short, almost complete exercise session when you are pressed for time. They are excellent for promoting overall flexibility, and help to prevent fat buildup, particularly at the midriff. A superb tension-reliever, they are also helpful in reducing stress.

Because the Sun Salutations encourage concentration and conscious breathing, they are a splendid set of exercises for promoting a 'fine-tuning-in' to yourself, so you can be more alert to departures from normal functioning. They also enhance vitality.

The Sun Salutations are beneficial to the lymphatic system (part of the immune system which protects you from disease). By contracting various muscles, the exercises exert gentle pressure on underlying blood and lymphatic vessels. The non-strenuous stretching action provided by the different movements temporarily removes 'kinks' from lymphatic vessels and promotes a smoother flow of lymph, which eliminates waste matter from the body.

1   Stand tall, with the palms of your hands together in front of your chest (Figure 26). Breathe regularly.
2   Inhale, raise your arms and carefully bend backwards to stretch the front of your body (Figure 27). Tighten your buttock muscles to help protect your lower back.
3   Exhaling, bend forwards (at your hip joints rather than your waist) and place your hands on the mat beside your feet (Figure 28). If necessary, bend your knees; as you become more flexible, you will be able to do this step with your knees straight.
4   Inhale and look up. Taking the weight of your body on both hands, step back with your left foot (Figure 29).
5   Briefly suspending your breath (neither inhaling nor exhaling), step backwards with your right foot. The weight of your body is now borne by your hands and feet, and your body is relatively level from the back of your head to your heels (Figure 30). This

is another version of the Inclined Plane (see page 90).

6   Exhale and lower your knees to the mat. Also lower your chin or forehead (whichever is more comfortable) and chest to the mat. Relax your feet (Figure 31). This is known as the 'knee-chest' position.

7   Inhaling, lower your body to the mat and slowly and carefully arch your back. Keep your head up and back, and your hands pressed to the mat. Also keep your pelvis on the mat. This is the same as the Cobra posture (see page 89) (Figure 32).

8   Exhale and point your toes forwards; push against the mat with your hands to help to raise your hips. Arms are straight (or almost straight), and your head hangs down. Aim your heels towards the mat but do not strain (Figure 33). This is the same as the Dog Stretch posture (see page 98).

9   Inhaling, look up, rock forwards onto your toes and step between your hands with your left foot (Figure 34).

10 Exhaling, step between your hands with your right foot and bend forwards, as in step 3 of these instructions (Figure 35).

11 Inhaling, come up carefully into an upright standing position, and move slowly into a backwards bend, as in step 2 of these instructions (Figure 36).

12 Exhaling, resume your starting position, as in step 1 of these instructions. Breathe regularly (Figure 37).

Repeat the entire sequence (steps 2 to 12) as many times as you wish, alternating your left foot with your right in steps 4 and 9. Rest afterwards.

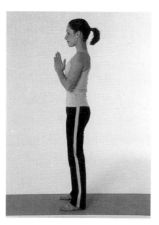

Fig. 26.
Sun Salutations:
Starting position

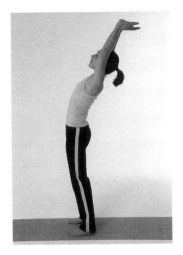

Fig. 27.
Sun Salutations:
Backwards stretch

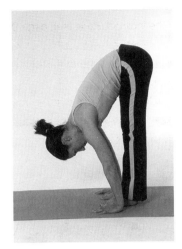

Fig. 28.
Sun Salutations:
Forwards bend, standing

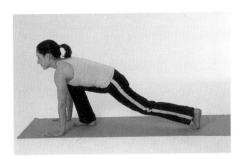

Fig. 29.
Sun Salutations:
Left leg stretch backwards

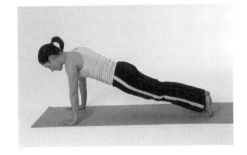

Fig. 30.
Sun Salutations:
Both legs back; body level

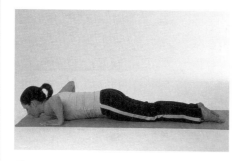

Fig. 31.
Sun Salutations:
'Knee-chest' position

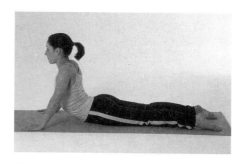

Fig. 32.
Sun Salutations:
Cobra

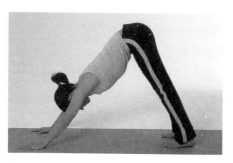

Fig. 33.
Sun Salutations:
Dog Stretch

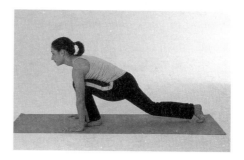

Fig. 34.
Sun Salutations:
Left leg forwards

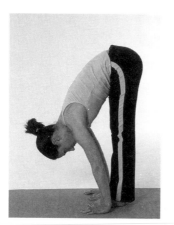

Fig. 35.
Sun Salutations:
Forward bend, standing

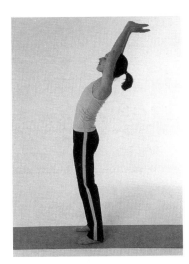

Fig. 36.
Sun Salutations:
Backwards stretch

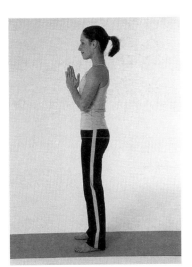

Fig. 37.
Sun Salutations:
Starting position

Cooling Down

Cooling down after exercise gives you an opportunity for static muscle stretching, which enhances your flexibility. It also allows your cardiovascular system (heart and blood vessels) to return gradually to normal functioning. In addition, it helps to prevent problems such as a sudden drop in blood pressure, feelings of light-headedness, dizziness, and fainting – any of which can occur if you stop exercising abruptly. A proper cool-down period after exercising, moreover, protects you against drastic temperature changes in the lungs, which can lead to broncho-constriction and induce asthma symptoms.

Done leisurely and consciously, all the warm-up exercises in this chapter (pages 45–59) can be used for cooling down. You may also add the Stick posture (see page 151) and the Rag Doll, which follows.

Rag Doll

1   Stand tall. Keep your arms at your sides. Relax your jaw and breathe regularly.
2   Tilt your head towards your chest, let your shoulders drop forwards and your arms
    and hands go limp (Figure 38).
3   Slowly curl your body forwards; let the weight of your arms pull you downward until
    your body hangs loosely, with your arms dangling (Figure 39). Imagine you are a floppy
    rag doll.
4   Stay in this posture as long as you are comfortable in it. Continue breathing regularly.
5   Slowly uncurl your body, from bottom to top, until you are again standing upright.
    Sit or lie down and rest.

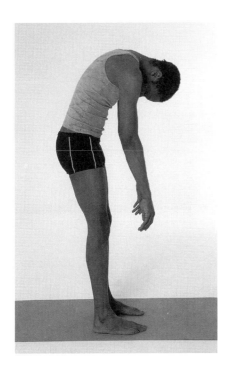

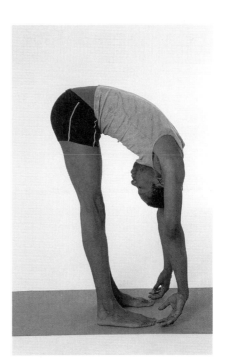

Fig. 38. Rag Doll:
Head down, shoulders drooping,
hands limp

Fig. 39. Rag Doll:
Completed posture

Posture

Postural patterns are influenced not only by your lifestyle but also by genetic and early environmental factors. Without conscious, sustained effort, faulty posture can become permanent.

The ideal posture for you is one in which your back is subjected to the least possible strain, and in which the normal graceful curves of the spine are maintained.

The key to good posture is fitness. If you keep your muscles well toned, you can acquire the posture that is right for you, especially if you complement this with a balanced mental and emotional state.

Good posture and freedom from the aches and pain generated by faulty posture can be acquired when all your muscles are used in accord with their anatomical function and the laws of body mechanics. The primary exercise for achieving these is the practice of correct postural habits during normal daily activities.

A well-aligned vertebral column when you are upright, or when you sit or lie down, imposes the least strain on the spine. It is also an important prerequisite for the harmonious functioning of the nervous system, which is hinged on the backbone and the spinal cord, and for the free expansion of the chest to facilitate unrestricted breathing.

In summary, your posture is determined by the way you hold each part of your body, from head to toe. It affects your breathing and indeed your overall health, physical and emotional. Your posture is also a reflection of the image you present to the world.

Following are five asanas that will help you to attain and maintain good posture and carriage.

Perfect Posture

CAUTION: Avoid this posture if you have varicose veins or venous blood clots, or if you experience any pain in your pubic area.

1   Sit comfortably with your legs outstretched in front of you.
2   Bend one leg and rest the sole of your foot against the opposite thigh, as far up as comfortable.
3   Bend the other leg and carefully place it in front of and against the opposite folded leg. Rest your hands on your knees or place them upturned in your lap (Figure 40).
4   You may change the position of your legs after a while, so that the one closer to your body is now in front.

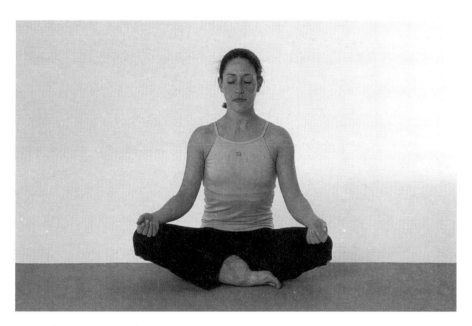

Fig. 40.
Perfect Posture

Firm Posture

CAUTION: Avoid this posture if you have varicose veins or venous blood clots, or if you experience pain in your pubic area.

1   Kneel down with your legs together and your body erect but not rigid. Point your feet backwards.
2   Slowly lower your body to sit on your heels. Rest your hands on your knees (Figure 41). Relax your jaw and breathe regularly.

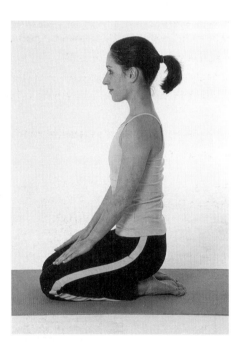

Fig. 41.
Firm Posture

Notes

This posture is also known as the Japanese Sitting Position.

If at first your heels cannot tolerate your weight, place a cushion or folded towel between your bottom and your heels, and maintain the posture for a short period only.

Posture Clasp

This posture is excellent for helping to prevent stiffness of the shoulder, arm and leg joints, and so keeping them flexible. It is also splendid for counteracting the effects of poor postural habits, and the aches that can result from activities that require much bending forwards.

1　Sit on your heels, Japanese style (see the Firm Posture, opposite). Relax your jaw and breathe regularly.
2　Reach over your left shoulder with your left hand. Keep your elbow pointing upwards rather than forwards, and your arm close to your ear.
3　With your right hand, reach behind your back from below, and interlock your fingers with those of your left hand. Maintain a naturally erect posture (Figure 42).
4　Stay in this posture as long as you comfortably can, breathing regularly.
5　Resume your starting position. Shrug your shoulders a few times or rotate them if you wish. Rest briefly.
6　Repeat steps 2 and 3, changing the position of your arms and hands (substitute the word 'left' for 'right' and vice versa in the instructions).

**Fig. 42.
Posture Clasp**

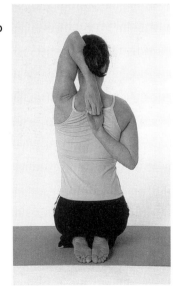

Notes

You can practice the Posture Clasp while standing, sitting on a stool, bench or other prop, or in a folded-legs posture. If you are unable to interlock your fingers, as described in step 3, use a scarf, belt or other suitable item as an extension to your arms. Toss one end over your shoulder and reach behind and below to grasp the other end. Pull upwards with your upper arm and downwards with your lower.

Chest Expander

The Chest Expander is superb for reducing a buildup of tension in your shoulders and upper back. Practice it periodically throughout your day at work or school, if you spend much time sitting at a desk or engaged in activities that require you to bend forwards a great deal. The Chest Expander also helps improve posture and facilitate unrestricted breathing, through which every body cell receives oxygen.

1   Stand tall with your feet comfortably apart and your arms at your sides. Relax your jaw and breathe regularly.
2   Inhale and swing your arms behind you; interlace the fingers of one hand with those of the other and raise your arms upwards to their comfortable limit. Maintain an upright posture (Figure 43), and keep breathing regularly.
3   Hold this posture for as long as you are comfortable in it.
4   Lower your arms, unlock your fingers and relax. You may shrug or rotate your shoulders a few times. Rest.

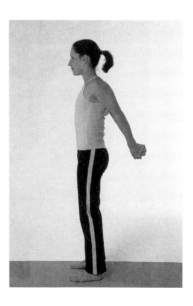

Fig. 43.
Chest Expander

You may practice the Chest Expander in any sitting position that permits free arm movement.

Mountain Posture

The Mountain Posture tones the pelvic, back and abdominal muscles and discourages fat deposits around the waist and abdomen. It improves muscular support of the viscera (internal organs). It also tones the chest and arm muscles and promotes deep breathing and good circulation.

1   Sit in any comfortable folded-legs posture, such as the Perfect Posture (page 63).
2   Inhale and stretch your arms overhead, keeping them close to your ears. Press your palms together if you can (Figure 44).
3   Hold this posture for as long as you comfortably can, breathing regularly.
4   Exhale, lower your arms and resume your starting position. Rest.

You may practice the Mountain Posture in any comfortable sitting position, or while sitting on a bench or stool.

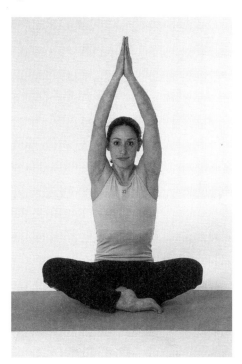

Fig. 44.
Mountain Posture

Abdominal Strengthening

Your abdominal muscles provide reinforcement for the muscles supporting your spine and pelvis. Weak abdominal muscles are a common cause of backache.

The four sets of abdominal muscles form a sort of corset spanning the front of the torso, from the breastbone and the ribs to the pubic bone, and around the side of the ridge of the pelvis, which some people can feel at the front of each hip.

Functions of the Abdominal Muscles
- To give support to the abdominal and pelvic organs, including the diaphragm.
- Along with the buttock muscles, to control the tilt of the pelvis, which influences good posture.
- To flex the trunk sideways; to raise it upwards from a supine (lying on the back) position; to help raise the legs while in a supine position; to rotate the trunk, and to help in bracing the body, as when lifting.
- To assist in conscious acts of breathing; in coughing, sneezing, shouting and singing; in eliminating wastes from the bladder and bowel, and also in the process of childbirth.

The following six asanas provide stretching and strengthening exercise for the four sets of muscles that make up the abdominal corset.

Yoga Sit-Up

1   Lie on your back, with your legs stretched out and slightly separated (Figure 45).

2   Bend your knees and slide your feet towards your bottom until the soles are flat on the mat. Maintain this distance between feet and bottom as you practice the sit-up. Rest your palms on your thighs (Figure 46).

3   Exhale as you slowly and carefully raise your head. Keep your gaze on your hands as you slide them towards your knees (Figure 47). When you feel the maximum tolerable tension in your abdomen, stop and hold the posture for as long as you are absolutely comfortable. Keep breathing regularly.

4   Inhale and resume your starting position by slowly curling your spine back onto the mat. Stretch out your legs, relax your arms at your sides, and rest.

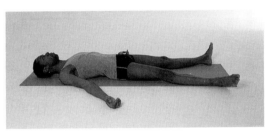

Fig. 45.
Yoga Sit-Up:
Starting position, lying on back

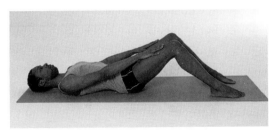

Fig. 46.
Yoga Sit-Up:
Legs bent, palms on thighs

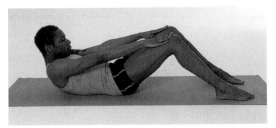

Fig. 47.
Yoga Sit-Up:
Completed posture

Physical Exercises

(Asanas)

Diagonal Curl-Up

1 Lie on your back, with your knees bent and the soles of your feet flat on the mat (Figure 48). Breathe regularly.

2 Slowly curl your upper body forwards, reaching with your hands towards the outside of your right knee (Figure 49). Synchronize your movement with regular breathing.

3 Hold this posture only as long as you are comfortable in it. Keep breathing regularly.

4 Slowly uncurl your body onto the mat; stretch out your legs, relax your arms at your sides and rest.

5 Repeat the Diagonal Curl-Up on the other side. Rest.

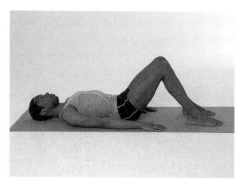

**Fig. 48.
Diagonal Curl-Up:
Starting position**

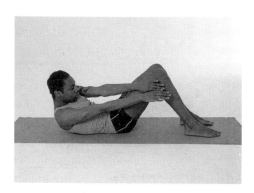

**Fig. 49.
Diagonal Curl-Up:
Completed posture, side view**

Angle Balance

1   Sit with your legs bent and the soles of your feet flat on the mat (Figure 50). Breathe regularly.

2   Tilt backwards so that you are balancing on your bottom; your feet are off the mat and your knees are closer to your chest (Figure 51). Focus your attention on your regular breathing to help you to maintain balance.

3   Stretch out your arms so that they are parallel to the mat. Also stretch out your legs (Figure 52). Keep focused, and adjust the degree of your tilt to assist you in keeping your balance.

4   Hold the posture as long as you comfortably can.

5   Resume your starting position. Rest.

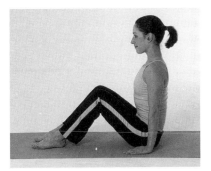

Fig. 50.
Angle Balance:
Sitting, knees bent, soles on mat

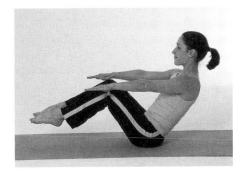

Fig. 51.
Angle Balance:
Feet off mat, body tilting back

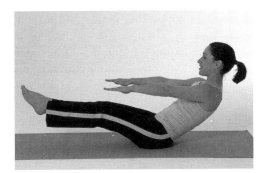

Fig. 52.
Angle Balance:
Completed posture, legs straight

Spinal Twist

1 Sit naturally erect on your mat, with your legs stretched out in front of you (Figure 53). Breathe regularly.

2 Bend your left leg and rest your left foot beside the outer aspect of your right knee.

3 On an exhalation, slowly and smoothly twist your upper body to the left and rest both hands on the mat on your left side. Turn your head and look over your left shoulder (Figure 54).

4 Hold the posture for as long as you comfortably can, breathing regularly.

5 Slowly untwist and return to your starting position. Rest briefly.

6 Repeat the twist, this time to the right as follows: Stretch your left leg in front of you. Bend your right leg. Place your right foot beside the outer aspect of your left knee. As you exhale, slowly and carefully twist your upper body to the right and place both hands on the mat at your right side. Turn your head and look over your right shoulder (Figure 55).

7 Slowly untwist, stretch out your legs and rest.

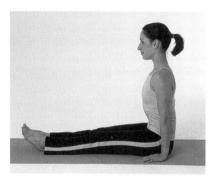

Fig. 53.
Spinal Twist:
Sitting, legs straight in front

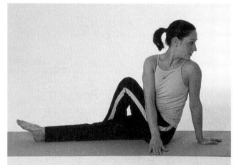

Fig. 54.
Spinal Twist:
To the left

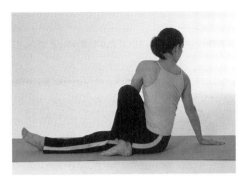

Fig. 55.
Spinal Twist:
To the right

Variation: Spinal Twist

1   Sit in a comfortable folded-legs posture. Hold on to your outer left thigh with your right
    hand. Slowly and carefully twist your upper body to your left. Rest your left hand on
    the mat behind you. Look over your left shoulder. Maintain regular breathing as you
    hold the posture as long as you comfortably can (Figure 56).

2   Slowly untwist your body. Rest briefly before repeating the twist to the right.

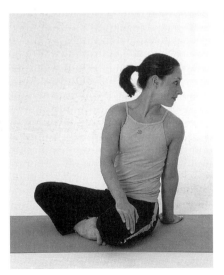

Fig. 56.
Spinal Twist variation:
Folded-legs posture

Physical Exercises

(Asanas)

Abdominal Lift

CAUTION: Do not practice this exercise if you have high blood pressure, an ulcer of the stomach or intestine (peptic ulcer), a heart problem or a hernia. Omit it during menstruation and pregnancy. In any case, check with your doctor before attempting this posture. Always practice it on an empty or near-empty stomach; never immediately after eating.

1   Stand with your feet about 25 centimeters (10 inches) apart. Bend your knees and turn them slightly outwards, as if preparing to sit.
2   Rest your hands on your thighs. Keep your torso as erect as you can and breathe regularly (Figure 57).
3   Exhale and with the air still expelled, briskly pull in your abdomen, as if to touch your spine with it, and also pull it upwards towards your ribs (Figure 58).
4   Hold the abdominal contraction until you feel the urge to inhale.
5   Inhale and straighten yourself. Rest briefly and resume normal breathing.
6   Repeat the exercise once, if you wish. You may also repeat it later.

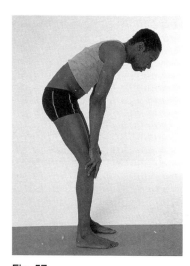

Fig. 57.
Abdominal Lift:
Starting position, side view

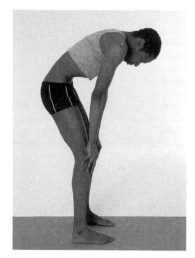

Fig. 58.
Abdominal Lift:
Abdomen pulled in on exhalation

Single Leg Raise

1   Lie on your back. Keep one leg stretched out straight in front, and the other bent with the sole of your foot on the mat. Relax your arms at your sides (Figure 59). Breathe regularly.

2   Press the small of your back to the mat. Exhale and raise the straight leg, slowly and with control, until it is about one-third vertical (Figure 60).

3   Hold the raised-leg posture as long as you comfortably can while breathing regularly.

4   Slowly and with control, lower the leg to the mat while inhaling. Rest briefly.

5   Repeat the exercise (steps 2 to 4), this time raising the other leg. Rest afterwards.

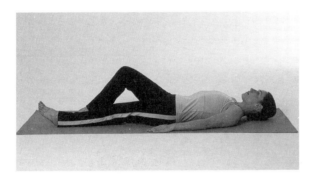

Fig. 59.
Single Leg Raise:
One leg bent, sole on mat,
other leg straight on mat

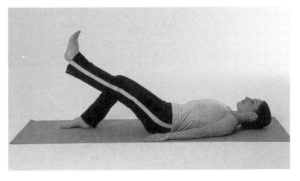

Fig. 60.
Single Leg Raise:
Straight leg raised about
one-third of vertical

Physical Exercises

(Asanas)

Forward-Bending (Back-Stretching) Postures

Apart from being complements to the backward-bending exercises (to follow), these forward-bending exercises promote the practice of diaphragmatic breathing (see pages 115–117). They also help the intercostal muscles (between the ribs) to become more mobile, and so counteract tension and rigidity. As you breathe rhythmically while maintaining (holding) these postures, your internal organs receive a gentle, therapeutic massage, which enhances circulation and facilitates the elimination of wastes.

Star Posture

1   Sit comfortably erect with your legs stretched out in front. Breathe regularly.
2   Fold one leg inwards and rest the sole of the foot beside the knee of the outstretched leg (Figure 61). This establishes the distance between the feet and the rest of the body once you are performing the exercise.
3   Fold the other leg and place the soles of the feet together (Figure 62).
4   Clasp your hands securely around your feet.
5   Exhaling, bend forwards slowly, smoothly and with control, bringing your face towards your feet. Once you have reached your comfortable limit, relax your head downwards (Figure 63).
6   Hold the posture for as long as you are comfortable in it while breathing regularly.
7   Slowly resume your starting position, synchronizing movement with breathing. Rest.

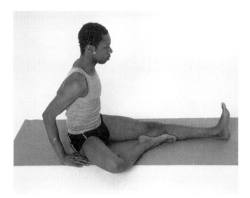

Fig. 61.
Star Posture:
Sitting, one leg straight,
other leg folded inwards

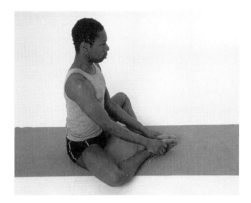

Fig. 62.
Star Posture:
Both legs folded inwards

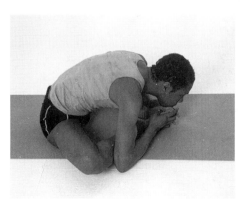

Fig. 63.
Star Posture:
Completed

Curling Leaf

1   Sit on your heels, Japanese style (Figure 64). Breathe regularly.

2   Slowly and carefully bend forwards. Rest your forehead on the mat (Figure 65), or turn it to the side. Relax your arms beside you.

3   Stay in this posture for as long as you are comfortable in it. Keep breathing regularly.

4   Slowly resume your starting position.

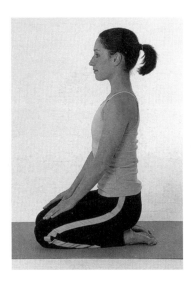

**Fig. 64.
Curling Leaf:
Starting position,
sitting on heels**

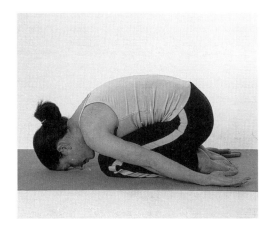

**Fig. 65.
Curling Leaf:
Completed posture**

Variation: Curling Leaf

Instead of resting your arms beside you, stretch them ahead of you (Figure 66).

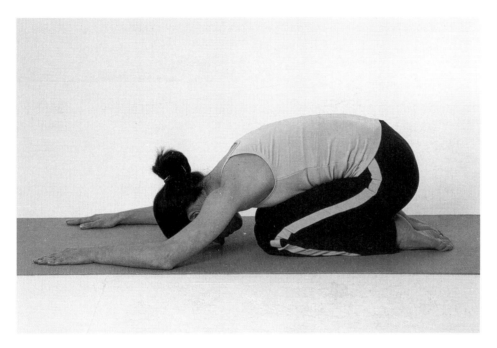

Fig. 66.
Curling Leaf variation:
Arms extended in front

Notes
This posture is also known as the Pose of a Child.

If you find it difficult for your head to reach the mat, place a cushion or pillow in front of you, on which to rest your forehead or face.

Single Knee Press

1 Lie on your back with your legs stretched out in front and your arms beside you.
2 Exhaling, bend one leg and bring the knee towards your chest. Clasp your hands around the bent knee (Figure 67).
3 Hold the posture for as long as you comfortably can while breathing regularly.
4 Inhale and release your hold on the leg; press the small of your back to the mat and lower your leg, slowly and with control.
5 Rest briefly and repeat the exercise (steps 2 to 4) with the other leg. Rest afterwards.

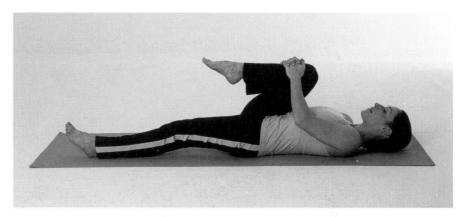

Fig. 67.
Single Knee Press

Backward-Bending Postures (Anterior Stretches)

Complementing the forward-bending exercises in the previous section are the following seven backward-bending postures, which stretch the front of the body. These postures are excellent for expanding the ribcage and so increasing the mobility of the chest wall. They thus facilitate deep, diaphragmatic breathing. They also help strengthen the back muscles and keep the spine flexible. In addition, they are beneficial to the functioning of endocrine glands, such as the thyroid and the adrenals.

The Bridge

1   Lie on your back with your legs bent and the soles of your feet flat on the mat,
    comfortably close to your bottom. Relax your arms beside you, with your palms turned
    downwards. Breathe regularly.
2   Inhaling, first raise your hips, then slowly and smoothly the rest of your back until your
    torso is fully raised (Figure 68). Do not arch the small of your back. Keep your feet,
    arms, hands, upper back and head in firm contact with the mat.
3   Hold the raised-torso posture as long as you comfortably can while breathing regularly.
4   Slowly and smoothly lower your torso, in reverse motion, as if curling your spine one
    bone at a time, onto the mat. Synchronize breathing with movement. Rest.

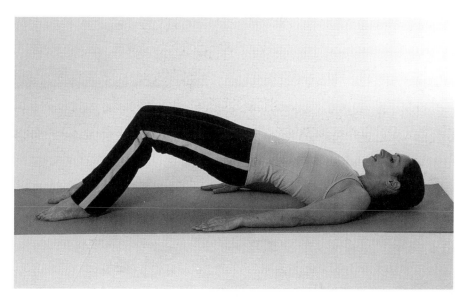

Fig. 68.
The Bridge

Variation: The Bridge

Follow the instructions for the basic Bridge posture, above, but this time stretch your arms overhead to their comfortable limit (Figure 69). Rest afterwards.

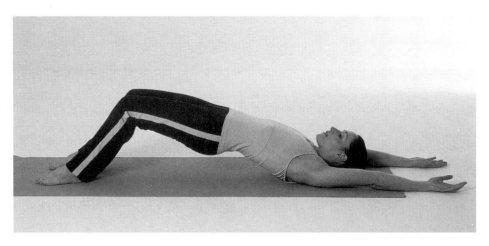

Fig. 69.
The Bridge variation:
Arms extended overhead

Fish Posture

CAUTION: Avoid this posture if you have an abdominal hernia or neck pain, or if you suffer from vertigo, dizziness, or balance disorders. Also avoid it during the first three days of menstruation, and check with your doctor if you have a thyroid gland problem and are considering practicing it.

1   Lie on your back with your legs stretched out in front and your arms beside you.
2   Bend your arms, push down on your elbows and raise your chest as you arch your back.
3   Carefully stretch your neck and ease your head towards your shoulders; rest the top of your head on the mat. Adjust your position so that most of your weight is taken by your bottom and elbows, rather than your head and neck (Figure 70).
4   Hold this posture for a few seconds to begin with, breathing slowly and as deeply as possible. Hold the posture longer when you feel more comfortable in it.
5   Slowly and carefully ease yourself out of the posture to resume your starting position. Rest.

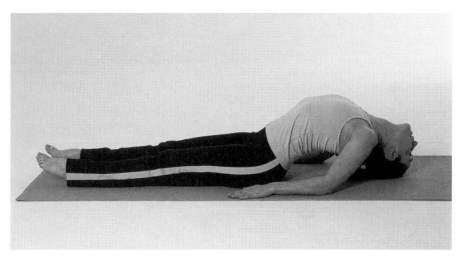

Fig. 70.
Fish Posture

Half Locust

CAUTION: Avoid the Half Locust if you have a serious heart condition or a hernia.

1   Lie on your abdomen, with your chin on the mat and your legs close together. Straighten your arms and position them, close together, under your body. Make fists and keep your thumbs down. (Alternatively, keep your arms by your body.) Breathe regularly.

2   Exhale and slowly and with control raise one still-straight leg as high as you comfortably can. Keep your chin, arms and body pressed to the mat (Figure 71).

3   Hold the raised-leg posture as long as you comfortably can while breathing regularly.

4   Lower your leg to the mat, slowly and with control. Rest briefly.

5   Repeat the exercise with your other leg. Rest.

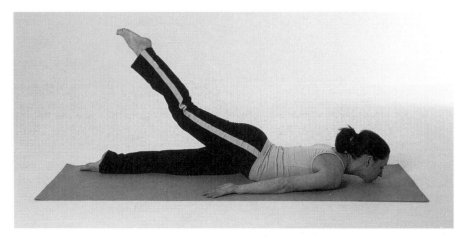

Fig. 71.
Half Locust

The Bow

CAUTION: Avoid this exercise if you have a serious heart condition or a hernia.

1   Lie face down, with your legs comfortably separated and your arms beside you (Figure 72). Breathe regularly.
2   Bend one leg and hold on to the foot, ankle or lower leg with the hand on the same side (Figure 73).
3   Bend the other leg and hold it, as in step 2 above (Figure 74).
4   Exhaling, push your feet upwards and away from you. This action will raise your legs and arch your body (Figure 75).
5   Hold this posture for as long as you comfortably can while breathing regularly.
6. Carefully resume your starting position. Rest.

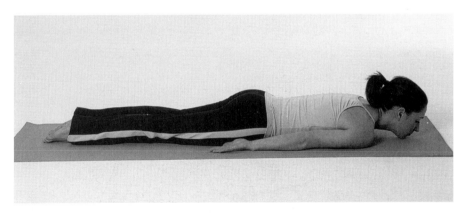

Fig. 72.
The Bow:
Starting position, lying face
downwards

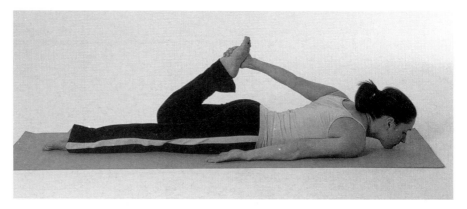

Fig. 73.
The Bow:
Lying face downwards,
one knee bent, hand holding foot,
ankle or lower leg

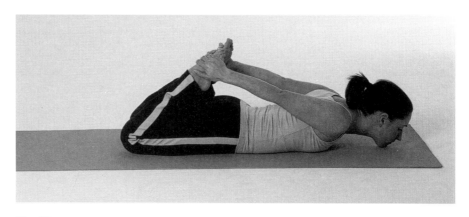

Fig. 74.
The Bow:
Lying face downwards,
both knees bent, hands holding feet,
ankles or lower legs

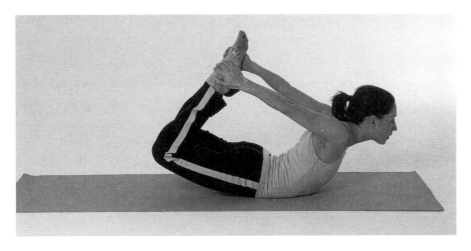

Fig. 75.
The Bow:
Completed posture

The Cobra

CAUTION: Do not practice the Cobra during pregnancy or if you have a hernia.

1   Lie on your abdomen, with your head turned to the side. Relax your arms and hands beside you. Breathe regularly.
2   Turn your head to the front and rest your forehead on the mat (Figure 76). Place your palms directly beneath your shoulders and keep your arms close to your sides.
3   On an inhalation, bend your neck backwards, slowly and carefully: touch the mat with your nose then your chin, in one smooth movement. Keep breathing regularly. Continue arching your spine: first the upper then the lower back (Figure 77), in one fluid movement.
4   When you can bend no farther with absolute comfort, hold the posture while breathing regularly. Keep your pelvis on the mat (Figure 78).
5   Come out of the posture in reverse, very slowly, smoothly and with control: lower your abdomen to the mat, then your chest, chin, nose and forehead, in synchronization with regular breathing.
6   Relax your arms beside you, turn your head to the side and rest (Figure 79).

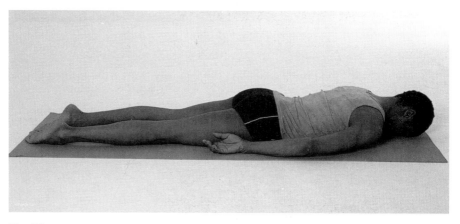

Fig. 76.
The Cobra:
Lying face downwards,
forehead on mat

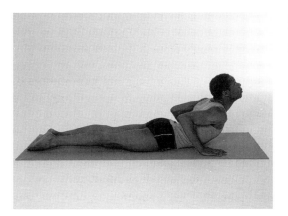

Fig.77.
The Cobra:
Midway position, back arched

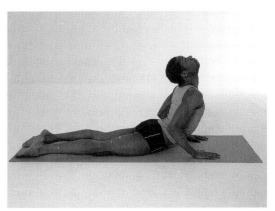

Fig. 78.
The Cobra:
Completed posture (keep pelvis
on mat)

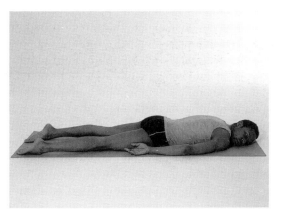

Fig. 79.
The Cobra:
Recovery, lying on abdomen,
face turned to the side

Inclined Plane

1   Sit tall, with your legs together and stretched out in front. Rest your hands on the
mat behind you, with your fingers pointing away from you. Keep your arms close to
your body. Breathe regularly (Figure 80).

2   Press your palms on the mat to help you to raise your body. Keep your hips high.
Carefully tilt your head back. Your body should be level from top to toes. Your weight
should be borne by your palms and feet (or heels) (Figure 81).

3   Hold the posture for as long as you are comfortable in it, breathing regularly.

4   Carefully bring your head up, lower your body to the mat and resume your starting
position. Relax your arms and hands and rest.

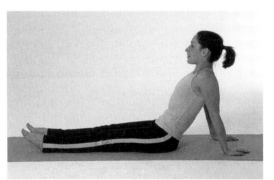

Fig. 80.
Inclined Plane:
Starting position – sitting
upright, legs together and
extended in front; hands on
mat, behind hips; fingers
pointing backwards;
arms close to body

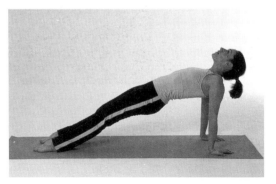

Fig. 81.
Inclined Plane:
Completed posture – body in
straight line from neck to foot

The Camel

CAUTION: Avoid this posture if you suffer from neck pain or spinal disc problems, or if you have a hernia.

1   Kneel down with your legs together and your toes pointing backwards (Figure 82).
2   Support the small of your back (waist level) with your hands, and very carefully tilt your head back.
3   Slowly and carefully place your right hand on your right heel and your left hand on your left heel. Keep your hips high (Figure 83).
4   Hold the posture for as long as you can with absolute comfort, breathing regularly.
5   Very slowly and carefully, resume your starting position. Rest.

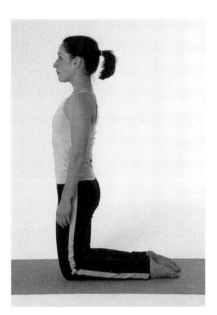

Fig. 82.
The Camel:
Starting position (kneeling upright)

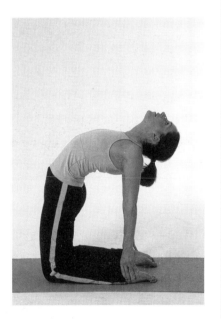

Fig. 83.
The Camel:
Completed posture

Sideways Stretches

Sideways-bending postures complement abdominal and backwards- and forwards-bending exercises. They thus contribute to the health of the spine, and they also discourage a buildup of excess weight at the midriff. This facilitates free diaphragmatic action and deep breathing. These exercises also enhance abdominal and pelvic circulation.

Half Moon

1   Stand naturally erect, with your feet close together and your body weight equally distributed between them. Relax your arms at your sides. Breathe regularly.
2   Inhale and raise your arms overhead. Press your palms together if you can (Figure 84). Keep your arms alongside your ears.
3   Exhale and slowly and smoothly bend your torso to one side to form a graceful arch (Figure 85).
4   Hold the posture for as long as you are comfortable in it while breathing regularly.
5   Resume your upright, starting position. Rest briefly.
6   Slowly and smoothly bend your torso to the other side, as in step 3.
7   Hold the posture for as long as you are comfortable in it while breathing regularly.
8   Resume your starting position. Rest.

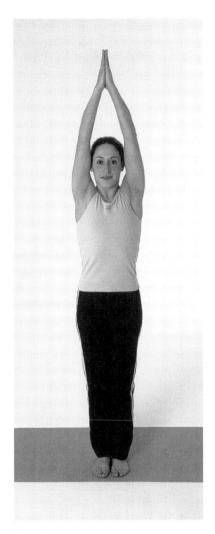

Fig. 84.
Half Moon:
Starting position –
arms overhead and straight,
palms together

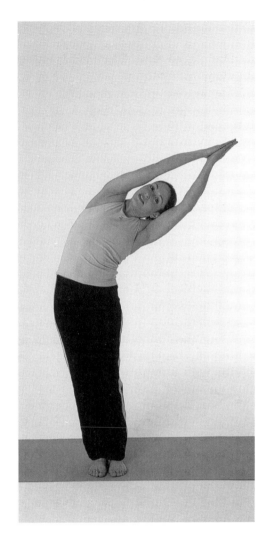

Fig. 85.
Half Moon:
Completed posture –
graceful sideways arch

Sideways Stretch in Sitting Folded-Legs Posture

1   Sit in any comfortable folded-legs posture, such as the Perfect Posture (see page 63). Breathe regularly.

2   Rest the palm of one hand on the mat beside your hip, with your fingers pointing forwards.

3   Exhaling, raise the other arm overhead and slowly and smoothly bend your upper body sideways, towards the hand on the mat (Figure 86). Keep the upper arm lined up with the ear to ensure a sideways rather than a forwards bend.

4   Hold the posture for as long as you comfortably can while breathing regularly.

5   Inhale and resume your starting position. Rest briefly.

6   Repeat the exercise on the other side (steps 2 to 5).

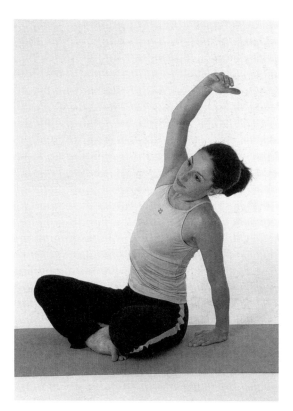

Fig. 86.
Sideways Stretch:
In sitting folded-legs posture,
completed

Angle Posture

1   Stand tall, with your arms at your sides and your feet about 60 centimeters (24 inches) apart. Breathe regularly.
2   Inhaling, raise your left arm. Exhaling, bend sideways to the right (Figure 87). As you do so, your right hand will slide down your leg. Keep your left arm alongside your ear.
3   When you can bend no farther, hold the posture for as long as you comfortably can while breathing regularly.
4   Inhale and resume your upright position. Exhale and lower your arm. Rest briefly.
5   Repeat the sideways bend to the other side (substitute the word 'right' for 'left' and vice versa in the instructions).

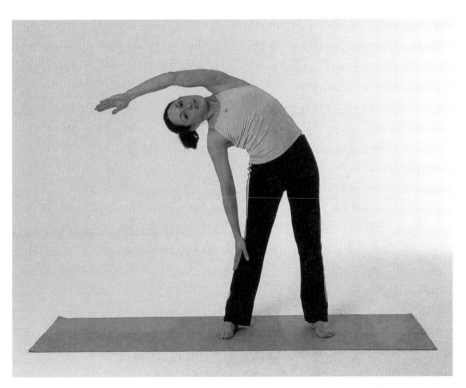

Fig. 87.
Angle Posture

Cross Beam

1 Kneel on your mat. Breathe regularly.

2 Stretch your right leg out to the side; point your toes towards the front rather than sideways, to prevent you from going into a 'split' as you do the posture.

3 Raise your left arm overhead, keeping it aligned with your ear. Rest your right hand on your right leg (Figure 88). Turn the palm upwards.

4 Exhale and bend to the right. As you do so, your right hand will slide down the leg (Figure 89). Keep your left shoulder back, to ensure a sideways rather than a forwards bend.

5 Hold the posture for as long as you comfortably can while breathing regularly.

6 Resume your starting position slowly, synchronizing movement with regular breathing. Rest briefly.

7 Repeat the sideways bend on the other side (steps 2 to 6); substitute the word 'left' for 'right' and vice versa in the instructions.

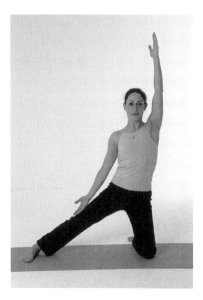

Fig. 88.
Cross Beam:
Starting position

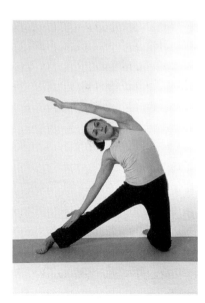

Fig. 89.
Cross Beam:
Completed posture

Inverted Postures

Useful in helping to drain mucus from the airways, thus relieving congestion in the lungs, these hips-high, head-low postures also enhance the functioning of organs and glands within the trunk, and improve circulation.

The Dog Stretch (Figure 91, page 98 and Figure 33, page 58) offers an additional benefit: it helps to maintain the elasticity of the hamstring muscles (hamstrings), which are at the back of the legs. When these shorten, they affect the tilt of the pelvis, which influences posture. Shortened hamstrings increase the arch of the spine at the lower back, and so impose strain on the back muscles.

Dog Stretch

CAUTIONS: Omit the Dog Stretch if you suffer from high blood pressure or have a heart condition or any disorder that produces feelings of light-headedness or dizziness when you hang your head down. See also the Half Shoulderstand (page 99) and the Full Shoulderstand (page 101) for other cautions related to inverted postures.

1 Start in an all-fours position on your hands and knees. Let your arms slope forwards and keep your back level (Figure 90). Breathe regularly.
2 Tuck your toes in so that they point forwards. Rock backwards slightly; raise your knees and straighten your legs. Straighten your arms. Look down. You are now in a hips-high, head-low posture (Figure 91). Aim your heels towards the mat but do not strain the muscles at the back of your legs.
3 Hold the posture for as long as you are comfortable in it, while breathing regularly.
4 Rock forwards gently and prepare to resume your starting position: sit on your heels in the Firm Posture (Figure 92).
5 Rest in the Curling Leaf posture (Figure 93).

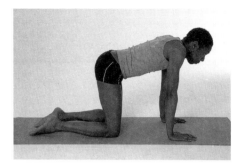

Fig. 90.
Dog Stretch:
Starting position on all fours,
back level

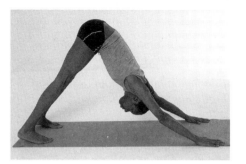

Fig. 91.
Dog Stretch:
Completed posture,
legs straight

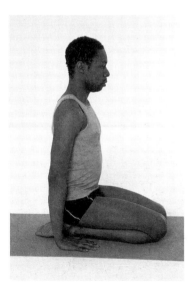

Fig. 92.
Dog Stretch:
Recovery in Firm Posture

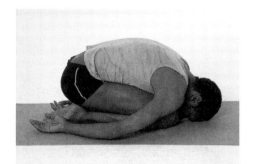

Fig. 93.
Dog Stretch:
Recovery in Curling Leaf posture

Half Shoulderstand

CAUTIONS: Avoid this and other inverted postures if you have an ear or eye disorder, or if you suffer from heart disease, high blood pressure or other circulatory disorder. Do not practice inverted postures during menstruation. In any event, check with your doctor before attempting the Half Shoulderstand and other head-low hips-high postures.

1   Lie on your back. Bend your knees and rest the soles of your feet flat on the mat. Keep your arms close to your sides (Figure 94). Breathe regularly throughout the exercise.
2   Bring first one knee, then the other, to your chest (Figure 95).
3   Straighten one leg at a time until your feet point upwards (Figure 96).
4   Kick backwards with both feet at once, until your hips are off the mat. Support your hips with your hands, thumbs in front (Figure 97).
5   Maintain the posture for a few seconds to begin with; longer as you become more comfortable with it.
6   To come out of the posture, rest your hands on the mat, close to your body. Keep your head pressed firmly to the mat (you may tilt your chin slightly upwards), and slowly and carefully lower your torso, from top to bottom, onto the mat. Bend your knees and stretch out your legs, one at a time. Rest.

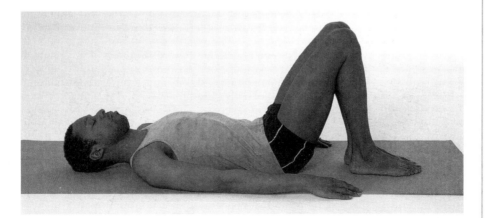

Fig. 94.
Half Shoulderstand: Starting position

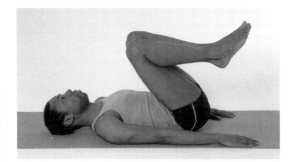

Fig. 95.
Half Shoulderstand:
Knees bent and brought
towards chest

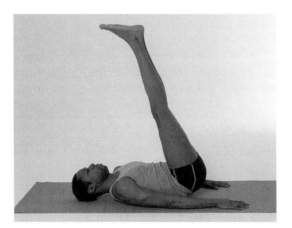

Fig. 96.
Half Shoulderstand:
Knees straightened

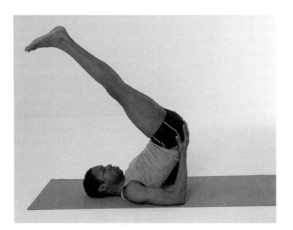

Fig. 97.
Half Shoulderstand:
Completed posture
(support hips with
hands)

Full Shoulderstand

CAUTIONS: These are the same as for the Half Shoulderstand (page 99). Avoid the Full Shoulderstand if you suffer from neck pain.

1   Lie on your back. Bend your knees and rest the soles of your feet flat on the mat. Keep your arms close to your sides. Breathe regularly throughout the exercise.
2   Bring first one knee, then the other, towards your chest.
3   Straighten one leg at a time until your feet point upwards.
4   Kick backwards with both feet at once, until your hips are off the mat. Support your hips with your hands, thumbs in front.
5   Gradually move your hands, one at a time, towards your upper back, until your body is in as vertical a position as you can manage with complete comfort. Your chin should be in contact with your chest, and your body as relaxed as possible (Figure 98).
6   Hold the posture for a few seconds to begin with, working up to two or more minutes as you become more accustomed to it.
7   To come out of the posture, tilt your feet slightly backwards. Rest your arms beside your body and keep your head pressed to the mat. Slowly lower your hips to the mat. Bend your legs and lower them, one at a time, to the mat. Rest.

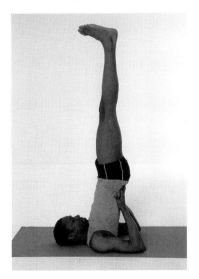

Fig. 98.
Full Shoulderstand:
Completed posture

Mock Headstand

CAUTION: If you have high blood pressure or neck pain, check with your doctor before practicing this posture.

1   Sit on your heels, with your toes pointing backwards. Breathe regularly throughout the exercise.
2   Lean forwards and rest your forehead on the mat, close to your knees (Figure 99).
3   Carefully raise your bottom from your heels, until the top of your head rests on the mat. Do not place pressure on your skull. Hold on to your ankles or heels (Figure 100).
4   Hold the posture for only a few seconds at first, working up to a minute or two as you become more comfortable in it.
5   To come out of the posture, ease yourself slowly towards your heels. Keep your head low for a few seconds before gradually sitting upright on your heels. Rest before getting up.

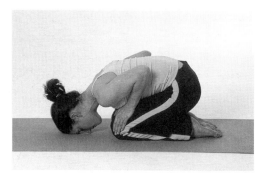

**Fig. 99.
Mock Headstand:
Starting position**

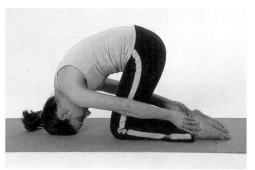

**Fig. 100.
Mock Headstand:
Completed**

Balance Postures

Balance postures train you to be focused by diverting your attention from environmental stimuli, many of which can be disturbing. They thus promote a sense of steadiness and calm, attributes which are useful in counteracting apprehension and anxiety. They are also excellent for cultivating nerve-muscle coordination, alertness and nerve control.

The Holy Fig Tree posture (Figure 114, page 111) offers the added benefits of boosting energy, improving circulation, and helping keep respiratory passages clear.

The Tree

1. Stand tall, with your feet close together and parallel to each other. Bring your hands together in front of your chest, in 'prayer position'. Breathe regularly.
2. Lift one leg and place the sole of your foot against the inner aspect of your opposite thigh (use your hands to help, if necessary) (Figure 101).
3. Hold the posture for as long as you can, breathing regularly and focusing your attention on your breathing to help you to stay steady. (You may also gaze at a still object to help you to maintain your balance.)
4. When you are ready to come out of the posture, straighten your bent leg and resume your starting position. Relax your hands at your sides. Rest briefly.
5. Repeat the exercise, balancing this time on the other foot.

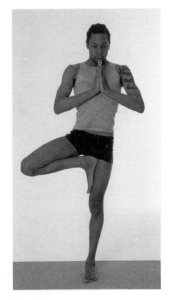

Fig. 101.
The Tree

Variation: The Tree

Instead of having your hands in front of your chest, as in step 1 above, raise your arms straight overhead and press your palms together, if you can (Figure 102).

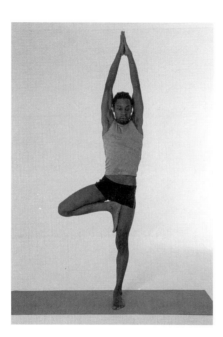

Fig. 102.
The Tree variation:
Arms overhead, palms together

The Stork

1   Stand tall, with your feet together. Breathe regularly.

2   Shift your weight onto one foot. Bend the other leg and point your foot backwards. Raise your arms at your sides; relax your wrists (Figure 103).

3   Imagine that you are a stork standing on one leg. Your arms are your wings. Hold the posture as long as you can while breathing regularly. Fix your attention on a still object, such as a picture on a wall, to help you to maintain balance.

4   Resume your starting position. Rest briefly.

5   Repeat the exercise (steps 2 to 4), this time bending the other leg. Rest afterwards.

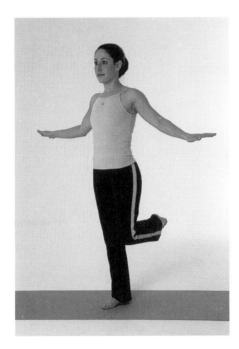

Fig. 103.
The Stork

Dancer's Pose

1   Stand tall, with your feet a little apart and your body weight equally distributed between them. Breathe regularly.

2   Shift your weight onto one foot. Bend your other leg, hold on to the foot and bring it close to your bottom. Raise your opposite arm straight upwards (Figure 104).

3   Hold the posture for as long as you can, focusing on your regular breathing to help you to stay steady.

4   Resume your starting position. Rest briefly.

5   Repeat the exercise (steps 2 to 4), this time balancing on the other foot. Rest afterwards.

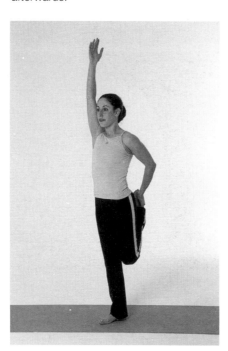

Fig. 104.
Dancer's Pose

Variation: Dancer's Pose

1 After completing the basic posture, as described above, slowly and carefully bend forwards. Still holding the foot of the bent leg, push it away from your bottom (Figure 105).

2 Hold the posture as long as you can. Resume your starting position and rest.

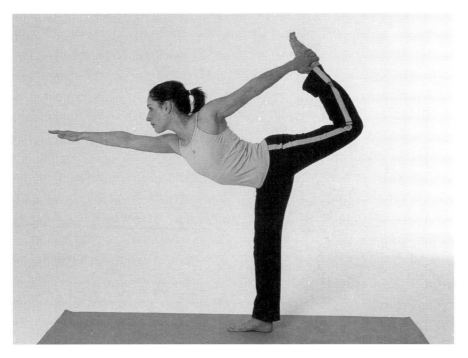

Fig. 105.
Dancer's Pose variation

The Eagle

1. Stand tall. Relax your arms at your sides. Keep your eyes open and breathe regularly.
2. Slowly lift your right leg. Do so with awareness so as to maintain your balance.
3. Cross your right leg over your left and hook your toes around your left lower leg. Adjust your posture to facilitate these movements.
4. When your stance is secure, straighten your body without putting unnecessary pressure on your left leg.
5. Now bend your right arm and position it in front of you, keeping your vision unobstructed.
6. Bend your left arm and place it within your bent right arm; rotate your wrists to bring your palms together (Figure 106).
7. Hold this posture as long as you can, focusing your attention on your regular breathing to help you to maintain balance.
8. When ready to come out of the posture, do so slowly and with awareness. Rest briefly.
9. Repeat steps 2 to 8, balancing on the right foot this time, and changing the position of the arms. Rest.

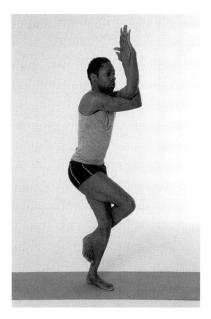

Fig. 106.
The Eagle

Toe-Finger Posture

1 Stand tall, with your weight equally distributed between your feet and your arms at your sides (Figure 107).
2 Shift your weight onto one foot. Slowly and carefully raise the other foot (Figure 108).
3 Grasp the toes of the raised foot (Figure 109). Focus on your regular breathing to help to keep you steady.
4 Keeping a secure hold on your toes, carefully straighten the raised leg (Figure 110).
5 Hold the posture for as long as you can while breathing regularly.
6 Carefully resume your starting position. Rest briefly.
7 Repeat the exercise (steps 2 to 6) with the other leg. Rest.

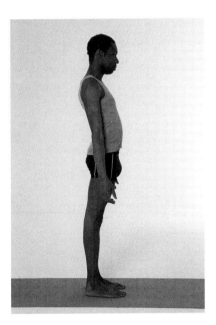

Fig. 107.
Toe-Finger Posture:
Starting position

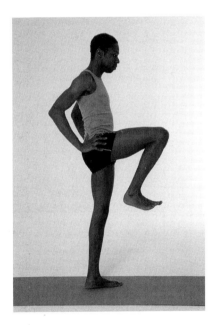

Fig. 108.
Toe-Finger Posture:
One leg lifted, knee bent

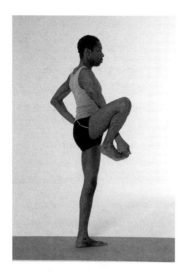

Fig. 109.
Toe-Finger Posture: Toes held

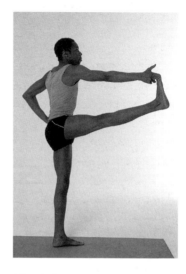

Fig. 110.
Toe-Finger Posture: Completed

Variation:
Toe-Finger Posture

1 Follow the instructions for the basic posture,
  as described above, then slowly
  and carefully bring your leg to the side, as far
  as you can with absolute comfort
  (Figure 111).
2 Hold the posture as long as you are
  comfortable in it, then resume your starting
  position and rest afterwards.

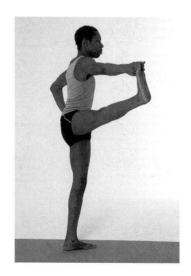

Fig. 111.
Toe-Finger Posture variation:
Leg to the side

Holy Fig Tree Posture

1 Stand tall and breathe regularly.
2 Raise your right arm straight overhead. Keep the arm aligned with the ear (Figure 112).
3 Raise your left arm to shoulder level; keep it straight (Figure 113).
4 Shift your weight onto your right foot and stretch your left leg backwards (Figure 114).
5 Hold the posture as long as you can while breathing regularly.
6 Repeat the exercise (steps 2 to 4), substituting the word 'right' for 'left' and vice versa in the instructions. Rest.

Remember to focus your attention on your regular breathing, or on a still object in front of you, to help you to maintain your balance.

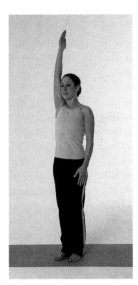 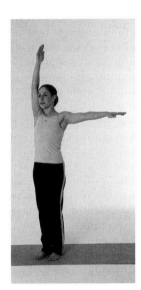 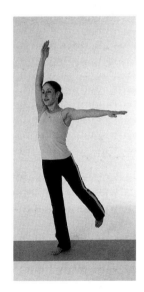

Fig. 112.
Holy Fig Tree Posture:
Right arm raised
straight overhead

Fig. 113.
Holy Fig Tree Posture:
Left arm stretched
sideways at shoulder
level

Fig. 114.
Holy Fig Tree Posture:
Completed (left leg
stretched backwards)

Breathing Exercises
(Pranayama)

Yoga breathing exercises are known collectively as *pranayama*. *Prana* means breath, vitality or energy, and *ayama* means stretching or expansion. Pranayama thus signifies the extension and control of breath, or voluntary controlled respiration. It is, in essence, the science of breathing, without which life ceases.

Benefits

By regularly practicing yoga breathing exercises, you can increase your potential for living to the fullest extent, instead of merely existing. You learn to become more aware, more alert, and more in control of yourself. This last point is a source of confidence and comfort in situations where one would otherwise feel at the mercy of outside forces.

Yoga breathing exercises strengthen your respiratory system, soothe your nervous system, and help eliminate various cravings (such as for nicotine, alcohol, and food). They also help fortify your immune system.

Breathing plays an important role in metabolism – the process by which the body utilizes nutrients. When practiced regularly, breathing exercises have a normalizing effect on both body weight and energy levels – two important considerations for people who tend to have breathing difficulties.

Because they improve the oxygen supply to all tissues, breathing exercises also enhance the functioning of all body structures. They help eliminate irritants that contribute to discomfort, pain, and difficulty breathing. They also retrain the muscles involved in the breathing process (see page 9), particularly the diaphragm. This improves the venous return of blood to your heart (see Figure 8, page 13) so that its workload is reduced and circulation is improved.

By consciously regulating your breath, you can help ease a troubled mind and stabilize your emotions. When your mind is uneasy, both your breathing and your heart rate tend to accelerate.

Prerequisites for Efficient Breathing

Awareness of the following key points will enable you to understand and master effective breath control:

1   A naturally erect posture/positioning of your vertebral column (spine), with your ribcage relaxed, avoids compressing your lungs and other vital structures within your chest (such as your heart and large blood vessels).
2   Slow, smooth, gentle movement of air when breathing requires less effort than fast, forceful breathing. It conserves energy and prevents fatigue. It also reduces the necessity to use accessory breathing muscles (such as those of the neck and shoulders), which usually come into play when breathing quickly, and which also requires harder work.
3   Unless otherwise specified in the exercise instructions, breathing through your nose, with your mouth closed, allows the air to be filtered, warmed, and moistened before it reaches the lungs.
4   A relaxed abdomen permits free and easy expansion during inhalation.
5   You want to achieve a slow, smooth, deep inhalation (without strain), first using your diaphragm like a suction pump and then expanding your ribcage with the help of your chest muscles. Similarly, effective breath control means practicing a slow, steady exhalation, using your diaphragm in reverse, as a sort of squeezing

pump. Try to make your exhalation longer than your inhalation.

6 A regular breathing rhythm is key, as is a relaxed body (pay special attention to your jaw, tongue, face, and hands).

7 You need to slow down, developing an awareness of the pace at which you perform various activities. Pacing yourself will promote respiratory control and comfort.

Preparing for the Exercises

Before practicing the exercises, attend to personal hygiene: empty your bladder and possibly your bowel also. Cleanse your mouth and your tongue (see page 125). Do a nasal wash (page 125).

You may practice the breathing exercises about 15 minutes following the asanas described in Chapter 4. Lie down and relax afterwards. The Pose of Tranquility (Figure 128, page 156) is ideal for this purpose.

(See Chapter 3, pages 37-40) for directions regarding food, drink, and time and place to practice.

Avoid practicing yoga postures immediately after a session of breathing exercises.

Cautions

Do not practice the Bellows Breath (page 123) if you have a heart disorder, high blood pressure, epilepsy, an ear or eye problem, or a hernia. Do not practice it during menstruation or pregnancy.

Do not hold your breath except under the supervision of an experienced yoga teacher.

Please also review the general cautions in Chapter 3 (pages 36–37).

The Exercises

RHYTHMIC DIAPHRAGMATIC BREATHING

About 80 percent of the work of breathing is accomplished by the diaphragm. Poor use of the diaphragm in breathing is possibly at the root of a large number of health disorders.

The blood flow at the base of the lungs, near the bottom of the ribcage where the diaphragm is situated, is over a liter per minute. By contrast, the blood flow at the top of the lungs is less than a tenth of a liter. Most of us are utilizing only this smaller area of lung tissue because of the habitual shallowness of our breathing.

By learning and practicing rhythmic diaphragmatic breathing, you will be able to use your diaphragm more efficiently than you perhaps now do, with much benefit to your whole system. You will also be decreasing the use of your accessory breathing muscles (such as those of the neck and shoulders), and consequently easing the work of breathing itself.

Please take a few moments to review the structure and function of the diaphragm (pages 10–11).

Benefits
Important benefits of the regular practice of breathing diaphragmatically include:

- reduction in respiratory rate (and therefore heart rate)
- increase in tidal volume (the volume of air inspired and expired in one normal respiratory cycle, that is, inhalation and exhalation)

- increase in alveolar ventilation
- decrease in residual volume (the volume of air remaining in the lungs at the end of maximal respiration)
- increase in the ability to cough effectively
- increased exercise tolerance
- improved circulation: the up-and-down motion of the diaphragm gives a gentle massage to abdominal organs; this improved circulation to these organs helps them function more efficiently
- rhythmic diaphragmatic breathing is a very important tool for stress reduction; it promotes a natural, even flow of breath, which strengthens the nervous system and relaxes the body; it is, in fact, the most efficient method of breathing, since it uses a minimum of effort in return for the maximum intake of oxygen.

1   Lie at full length on your back, with a pillow, cushion or folded towel under your head. Close your eyes or keep them open. Relax your jaw and breathe regularly.
2   Rest one hand lightly on your abdomen, just beneath your breastbone. Rest the fingers of your other hand on your chest, just below the nipple (Figure 115).
3   Keeping your abdomen as relaxed as possible, inhale through your nose slowly, smoothly and as fully as you can without strain. As you do so, the hand on the abdomen should rise as the abdomen moves upwards (Figure 116). There should be little or no movement of the fingers resting on the chest.
4   Exhale through your nose slowly, smoothly and as completely as you can, without force. As you do so, the hand on the abdomen should move downwards as the abdomen contracts (tightens) (Figure 117).
5   Repeat steps 3 and 4 several times in smooth succession.
6   Relax your arms and hands. Breathe regularly.

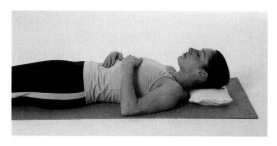

Fig. 115.
Rhythmic Diaphragmatic Breathing:
Starting position

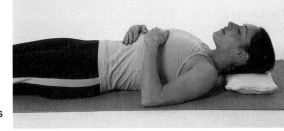

Fig. 116.
Rhythmic Diaphragmatic
Breathing:
Inhalation – abdomen rises

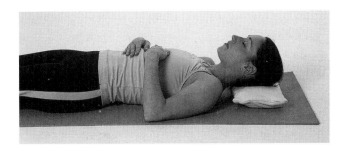

Fig. 117.
Rhythmic Diaphragmatic
Breathing:
Exhalation – abdomen
contracts (tightens)

Notes

- You may exhale through pursed lips, as if cooling a hot drink (see the Whispering Breath, page 144).
- If you begin to feel lightheaded, immediately resume your usual breathing. If you are standing, sit down.
- If in doubt whether your abdomen should rise or fall on inhalation, think of a balloon: as you put air into it, it becomes larger; when you let the air out, it becomes flat. The following mnemonic may be useful: 'Air in, abdomen fat; air out, abdomen flat.'
- If you find it difficult to coordinate inhalation with abdominal muscle relaxation, and exhalation with abdominal muscle contraction, place a light object, such as a small pillow, a plastic duck or boat, or a paper airplane on your abdomen to provide visual feedback.
- When you have mastered diaphragmatic breathing in a supine position, try it in other positions: semi-reclining, sitting or standing. Coordinate it with daily activities such as vacuum-cleaning, raking leaves, or walking up and down stairs.

Sandbag Breathing

The abdominal-strengthening exercises in Chapter 4 (pages 68–75) will condition your diaphragm and abdominal muscles. The breathing exercise that follows will further strengthen these structures.

To start, you will need a sandbag weighing approximately 1 lb (500 g). As your muscles become stronger and your breathing more efficient, you can increase the weight to a maximum of 10 lb (5 kg).

An alternative to a sandbag is a bag of rice or dried peas, beans or lentils. Be sure that the bag is sufficiently malleable to conform to your torso.

Practice Sandbag Breathing every day until you feel that your diaphragm and abdominal muscles are strong. You can then practice diaphragmatic breathing without a weight on your midriff.

1   Lie on your back. Place the sandbag (or bag of peas, etc.) on the middle of your torso, between your chest and abdomen. Comfortably separate your feet. Rest your outstretched arms beside you, a little away from your body. Relax, paying special attention to your jaw, facial muscles, and hands. Close your eyes or keep them open. Let your breath flow naturally (Figure 118).
2   Start breathing diaphragmatically: keeping your abdomen relaxed, inhale through your nose slowly, smoothly and as fully as you can without strain. As you do so, the sandbag should rise.
3   Exhale through your nose (or through pursed lips) slowly, smoothly, and as completely as you can without force. As you do so, the sandbag should descend.
4   Repeat steps 2 and 3 as many times as you wish in smooth succession.
5   Remove the sandbag. Breathe regularly.

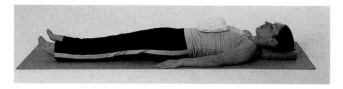

Fig. 118.
Sandbag Breathing

The Sniffing Breath

A counterpart of the Divided Breath (to follow), this exercise is excellent for relaxing a tight chest to facilitate deep breathing. Practice it any time you feel under pressure, to help you to relax and remain controlled.

1. Sit upright but not rigid, with the crown of your head uppermost. Relax your jaw. Breathe regularly. (You may also practice the Sniffing Breath while lying down or standing.)
2. Take two, three or more quick inward sniffs, as if breaking an inhalation into small parts.
3. Exhale slowly and steadily through your nose or through pursed lips.
4. Repeat steps 2 and 3 several times, until you feel your chest relaxing and you are able to take a deep inward breath without straining.
5. Resume regular breathing.

The Divided Breath

Because it helps empty the lungs completely, this exercise facilitates deep inhalation so that air can reach the bottom of your lungs where the exchange of gases takes place (see page 12).

The Divided Breath is also useful when you feel anxious or otherwise stressed, or have difficulty falling asleep or getting back to sleep.

1   Lie full length on your back. Close your eyes or keep them open. Relax your jaw and breathe regularly.
2   Inhale slowly, smoothly, and as fully as you can without strain.
3   To exhale, divide your breath into two, three or four roughly equal parts, with a brief pause between each. Make the last part smooth and sustained, without forcing it.
4   Repeat steps 2 and 3 several times in succession. The sequence is as follows:

Breathing Exercises

(Pranayama)

- slow, smooth inhalation
- one-third (or one-half or one-fourth) of an exhalation
- brief pause
- one-third (or one-half or one-fourth) of an exhalation
- brief pause
- complete the exhalation, sustaining the outgoing breath until there is a perceptible but gentle tightening of your abdomen.

5 Relax your abdomen and inhale. Resume regular breathing.

Notes
- Regular practice will help you avoid making the breath divisions or the pauses too long.
- Incorporate imagery of your choice into this exercise. You may, for example, use the mental picture of an elevator moving from floor to floor. Or you could visualize going down one step at a time, to correspond with each part of your exhalation.
- You may practice this exercise while sitting or standing.
- If necessary, take a few regular breaths after each exhalation has been completed, and then repeat the entire exercise.

Alternate Nostril Breathing

This exercise stimulates the inner lining of the nose by altering the air flow and sending sequential impulses to the two brain hemispheres.

Modern research has revealed that each of these two hemispheres has different functions: the left chiefly influences language and mathematical skills, while the right controls imaginative and intuitive functions such as spatial orientation and creative thinking.

Alternate Nostril Breathing helps to integrate the functioning of both hemispheres, which results in a harmonizing of mind and body, and also greater mental and physical energy. In addition, it is a very soothing and relaxing exercise. It helps counteract anxiety, which often accompanies asthma episodes, and which can also aggravate pain and other discomforts, both physical and emotional. Practicing Alternate Nostril Breathing is also a useful antidote for sleeplessness.

1   Sit tall in any comfortable position, with the crown of your head uppermost. Relax your body. Relax your jaw and breathe regularly.

2   Rest your left hand in your lap, on your knee or on the armrest of a chair, depending where you are seated.

3   Arrange the fingers of your right hand as follows: fold the two middle fingers towards your palm, or rest them lightly on the bridge of your nose; use your thumb to close your right nostril once the exercise is in progress, and use your ring finger (or ring and little fingers) to close your left nostril (Figure 119).

4   Close your eyes and begin: Close your right nostril and inhale slowly, smoothly, and as deeply as you can without strain, through your left nostril.

5   Close your left nostril and release your right nostril. Exhale.

6   Inhale through your right nostril.

7   Close your right nostril and release your left. Exhale. This completes one 'round' of Alternate Nostril Breathing (Figures 120 and 121).

8   Repeat steps 4 to 7 in smooth succession as many times as you wish.

9   Relax your right arm and hand. Resume regular breathing. Open your eyes.

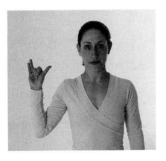

Fig. 119.
Alternate Nostril Breathing:
Showing arrangement of
fingers of right hand

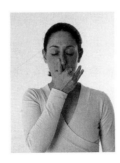

Fig. 120.
Alternate Nostril
Breathing

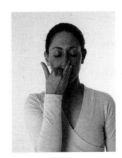

Fig. 121.
Alternate Nostril
Breathing

Notes

Always switch to the other nostril after the incoming breath; never after the outgoing breath.

If unable to sit upright, you may try this exercise in a semi-reclining or lying-down position, or even while standing.

Ujjayi Pranayama

The prefix 'ud' attached to nouns and verbs in the Sanskrit language implies a blowing or expanding. The word 'jaya' denotes victory or success, and implies restraint. Pranayama is the word used to describe yoga's breathing exercises. Ujjayi Pranayama is therefore also breath with sound, and is sometimes referred to as the Victorious Breath.

WHAT IT DOES

Vocalizing emotion through breath is one of Nature's outlets for the release of difficult sensations. Ujjayi Pranayama is one way to do this. It also improves the ventilation of the lungs, calms frayed nerves, and replenishes energy. It helps slow down the heart rate and so ease the heart's workload. It also contributes to strengthening the immune system, which protects the body from invasion of harmful organisms and infection.

As an introduction to this technique, imagine that you're blowing onto a window pane to make it foggy, by whispering the syllable 'haa'. This will help you bring about a relaxation of your throat, which is necessary for the correct execution of the breathing exercise itself. Now you are ready to begin.

1   Relax your jaw, keeping your lips closed though not compressed. Inhale slowly through your nose while pretending to say 'haa'.

2   Exhale slowly and completely through your nose, with your mouth still closed, while again mentally saying 'haa'.

3   Repeat steps 1 and 2 again and again, in smooth succession. Listen for a smooth, even sound which will indicate calm, in contrast with a rough, uneven one which suggests some agitation.

4   Resume regular breathing.

Notes

You may integrate visualization into this exercise. If you are familiar with the Star Wars movies, for example, you may pretend to be the character Darth Vader, whose breathing is reminiscent of Ujjayi Pranayama.

Bellows Breath

CAUTIONS: Do not practice this breathing exercise if you have any of the following disorders: a heart abnormality or high blood pressure; epilepsy, a hernia or an ear or eye problem; a herniated ('slipped') spinal disc. Do not practice it during menstruation or pregnancy.

Wait for two or three hours after eating to practice this exercise; never practice it immediately after having eaten.

WHAT IT DOES

Wonderful for thoroughly cleansing the sinuses and other respiratory passages, this exercise stimulates lung tissues and gently yet effectively massages abdominal organs. It thus helps improve the elimination of body wastes. In addition, the Bellows Breath is superb for strengthening the diaphragm and the abdominal muscles.

This exercise, in addition, provides excellent training in the voluntary control of exhalation, a skill those who suffer from respiratory disorders such as asthma will find useful. It also revitalizes the nervous system. Practice it when your energy begins to flag and you need to invigorate yourself.

1 Sit comfortably, with good posture. Relax your shoulders, arms and hands. Close your eyes or keep them open. Relax your jaw and breathe regularly.
2 Inhale slowly, smoothly, and as fully as you can without strain.
3 Exhale briskly through your nose as if sneezing, focusing your attention on your abdomen, which will tighten and flatten.
4 Inhalation will follow automatically as you relax your abdomen and chest.
5 Repeat steps 3 and 4 again and again in quick succession. Try to do so about six times to start with. Gradually increase the number of times as your stamina increases and you become more familiar with the technique.
6 Rest. Resume regular breathing.

Notes
- You may practice the Bellows Breath while standing.
- The abdominal action in this exercise, and also the sound of the breath as it is being performed, are reminiscent of the expanding and collapsing of a bellows as it drives a blast of air into a fire (it is, in fact, sometimes called the Breath of Fire).
- Visualizing this process may be useful in helping you to grasp and master the technique.
- Practice this exercise outdoors whenever you can, provided the air is relatively unpolluted.

On pages 143–144 you will read about hyperventilation (over-breathing), and you may wonder why you should practice an exercise that involves rapid breathing. The Bellows Breath differs from hyperventilation, however, in that it is done consciously and with your control, whereas hyperventilation is involuntary. The Bellows Breath results in thorough exhalation and, consequently, a full spontaneous inhalation. In hyperventilation, by contrast, the exhalation is fast and incomplete, and there's a sort of desperation for the next inhalation. Consequently, carbon dioxide stores are quickly depleted, producing the unpleasant effects of hyperventilation (see page 144). This does not occur when you practice the Bellows Breath.

Hygiene Practices

The Nasal Wash (Neti)
One safe and effective way of helping keep your nasal passages clear, and to soothe their mucous lining, is by means of a Nasal Wash, or *Neti*. This method also increases the tolerance of the lining to various irritants, and is a splendid treatment for sinus problems and allergic rhinitis, as occurs in disorders such as hay fever.

Being able to breathe freely through both nostrils is said to promote mental harmony. The Nasal Wash is therefore also useful prior to any meditation practice. Do it when preparing for a session of breathing exercises, or at any other time when you feel the need. Generally, up to three times a day is suggested.

1   Dissolve a quarter of a teaspoon of salt in 1 cup of warm water. (This is approximately the concentration of sodium [salt] in blood and tissue fluids.)
2   Pour a little of the salt-water solution into a clean cupped hand and carefully inhale some of it into one nostril, while closing the other nostril with a thumb or index finger.
3   Briskly, but not forcefully, breathe out to expel the liquid. Repeat the procedure.
4   Repeat the whole process with the other nostril.

Special *neti* pots are available for this procedure in stores that sell yoga supplies.

Tongue Cleansing
People with breathing difficulties tend to breathe through their mouth. Consequently, the membranes lining the mouth become dry and vulnerable to infection. Good oral hygiene, including daily tongue cleansing, is therefore suggested.

In addition to practicing the Lion (Figures 127 and 128, page 158), to exercise the tongue and keep it free of unnecessary tension, the practice of daily tongue cleansing is also beneficial. It helps, in addition, to keep your breath fresh, and is useful in averting a sore throat or preventing one from getting any worse.

You will need a metal teaspoon, reserved for this purpose only. (A toothbrush is not recommended. Special tongue-scrapers are also available in some health food stores and those specializing in hygiene and yoga supplies.)

1　Exhale and stick out your tongue. With the teaspoon inverted, gently scrape away, from back to front, deposits that have accumulated on your tongue. Rinse the spoon under cool running water.
2　Close your mouth and inhale.
3　Exhale and repeat the tongue cleansing (steps 1 and 2) once or twice.
4　Finish by thoroughly rinsing your mouth, and perhaps also flossing your teeth.
5　Clean the teaspoon with soap and water. Dry it and put it away for future use.

Comfort Measures

Controlled Coughing
Controlled coughing is a preventive measure to take against the explosive type of coughing that increases pressure within the chest, and which leads to airway collapse and blocks the effective removal of sputum. It is also less tiring and produces less wheezing. It helps, in addition, to move secretions from the smaller to the larger airways.

The technique to follow is sometimes called 'series', 'cascade' or 'staged' coughing, and it is an excellent means of clearing the airways and preventing infection. Moreover, it removes the fear of breathlessness, so that you can cough with confidence.

1　Sit on a chair, on a mat on the floor, or near the edge of a bed with your feet supported. Lean forwards slightly.
2　Take a few comfortably deep breaths, using the pursed-lip technique described in the Whispering Breath (see page 145).
3　Take a slow, deep inhalation through your nose, to increase lung volume and allow air to travel past the retained mucus.

4　Give three or four short coughs until there is little air remaining.

5　Repeat steps 2 to 4 as many times as you comfortably can.

6　Finish with a short period of deep diaphragmatic breathing through the nose or pursed lips.

7　Resume regular breathing.

Clearing the Airways

Chronic exposure to respiratory irritants can damage the natural cleaning system of the lungs. This system is composed of cilia and the mucous membranes from which they grow (see page 5). These membranes which line the airways continuously secrete mucus. The mucus is thin and sticky and helps to protect the lungs by trapping particles, such as dust, debris, and bacteria, not filtered by the nose.

The mucus moves constantly, carrying along everything caught in it, through the action of the untiring cilia. It eventually ends up in the intestinal tract, where digestive enzymes dissolve it and its contents.

When the airways become plugged with an increased quantity of mucus – a superb breeding ground for infection – here are steps to take to help clear the airways of sputum, and to keep them clear:

- Dilute the mucus, which tends to be thick, by increasing your intake of liquids such as plain water, warm water with lemon and honey, and also unsweetened fruit juices. Limit the tea, coffee and alcohol you drink, since these are diuretic and dehydrating.
- Use your prescribed broncho-dilator to relax the smooth muscles surrounding your bronchial tubes.
- Keep active: Go for a short walk or do a few minutes of gentle exercises. The warm-ups in Chapter 4 (pages 45–89) are appropriate.
- Do controlled coughing, as described above. This will move the mucus along and facilitate its expulsion.

Positions to Ease Breathlessness

You can minimize the effort of breathing and help prevent breathlessness by assuming certain positions that facilitate the work of the diaphragm. These positions are sometimes called 'dyspnea positions'. They permit maximum relaxation of the upper chest while allowing freedom of movement of the lower chest. If you are very short of breath, you may start with five or six breaths through your mouth before switching to diaphragmatic breathing through your nose or pursed lips, or a combination of the two.

Here are some suggested positions to ease difficult breathing:

- Arrange three or four pillows in a slope. Lie against them so that your upper body is raised and supported.
- Sit on a chair, bench or stool, or any other appropriate prop. Keep your torso as erect as possible without being rigid. Lean forwards and rest your forearms on your thighs; keep your wrists and hands relaxed.
- Sit near a desk, table, or other suitable prop. Keep your torso as erect as possible without being rigid. Lean forwards and rest your head on one, two or three stacked pillows or cushions placed on the prop. Rest your chest and shoulders against the pillows or cushions, and relax your arms beside them. This is a particularly useful position for sudden shortness of breath at night.
- Stand about a foot away from a wall, post, tree trunk, or other prop. Rest the lower half of your back against the prop. Relax your arms at your sides; relax your shoulders. This position and the one following are useful when you need to stop for a rest, almost anywhere.
- Keeping your back straight but not stiff, lean forwards and rest your forearms on any stable available prop, such as a banister, fence, or worktop.

The Pelvic Diaphragm

Apart from the respiratory diaphragm (see page 10), there is another, located between the legs, extending from the coccyx (tailbone) at the back to the pubic bone in front. Although situated somewhat remotely from the other diaphragm – which has been mentioned many times in this book so far – it nevertheless has a significant bearing on the efficiency with which we breathe.

The pelvic diaphragm is a sling-like muscular support for the pelvic organs, helping these structures withstand increases in pressure in the abdomen and pelvis, as occur when we cough, sneeze, or laugh. It plays an important part in respiration, since it markedly affects residual volume – that is, the volume of air remaining in the lungs at the end of maximal expiration.

Pelvic Floor Exercises

Exercises to strengthen the pelvic floor (lowest part of the torso) should be integrated into every program of breathing exercises. Apart from contributing to greater efficiency in breathing, they help to maintain good muscle tone and so prevent conditions such as hemorrhoids, uterine prolapse, and stress incontinence (in which urine escapes when abdominal pressure increases, as when you cough, sneeze, or laugh).

Perineal Exercise
One of the simplest and most effective pelvic floor exercises is the Perineal Exercise, and here's how to do it.

1. Sit, lie or stand comfortably. Relax your jaw and breathe regularly.
2. Exhale and tighten your perineum (tissues between the anus and external genitals).
3. Hold for as long as your exhalation lasts, but do not hold your breath.
4. Inhale and relax. Breathe regularly.
5. Repeat steps 2 to 4 once. Repeat regularly throughout the day.

Notes

- Practice the Perineal Exercise several times throughout the day. Practice it anywhere you wish: no one will know what you are doing.
- Avoid tensing your thigh muscles when practicing the exercise. Concentrate instead on tightening the perineal muscles themselves.
- Regular attempts at stopping and re-starting the flow of urine will give you practice in the action involved in the Perineal Exercise.

Mind Power

*As you ought not to attempt to cure the eyes without the head, or
the head without the body, so neither ought you to attempt to cure
the body without the soul ... for the part can never be well
unless the whole is well.*

PLATO

In the past when people were physically ill, they sought out a doctor for consultation and treatment. When mentally ill, they enlisted the help of a psychologist or psychiatrist. For a troubled spirit, the priest or other religious adviser was the therapist of choice.

Today, the enlightened are well aware of the inter-dependence of these three aspects of the human being. They also acknowledge that no one of them can suffer without involving the other two. Because we live in a society where we seem to need tangibles to explain effects, however, there are still those who are untrusting of results brought about by inner, intangible resources: that which we have within us and carry wherever we are, namely our feelings, our mental processes, and our breath. And yet there is a wealth of documented evidence to support the powerful influence that the mind has over the body. Awareness of this inter-connection can help asthma sufferers long-used to treating only their physical symptoms.

Psychoneuroimmunology (PNI)

A relatively new breed of specialists are helping to cast light on the mind–body connection. Their specialty is known as psychoneuroimmunology, or PNI. It refers to the interaction among three body systems: endocrine, nervous, and immune. PNI researchers investigate the way the brain affects the body's disease-fighting cells. They have found that the brain can transmit signals along nerve pathways to reinforce the body's defenses against infection. They have also demonstrated that this transmission of nerve signals can be controlled by thoughts and emotions.

By learning and practicing mind control you can, to some extent, influence hormonal activity – which, in turn, will have a regulating effect on your immune system. This skill can be used to complement any therapy you may be receiving for asthma or any health condition. You can use it to help stay well. Along with adequate nutritional support, regular exercise, and effective stress-reduction strategies, you can put this skill into practice to give yourself the best possible chance of attaining and maintaining optimum health.

Visualization

The ability to form pictures in your mind is known as visualization or imagery. It is not merely wishful thinking, and there is nothing magical about it. It is not the same as day-dreaming or fantasizing, both of which are passive and unfocused activities. Visualization is active and purposeful.

Over the past couple of decades, researchers' findings indicate that anyone can learn to control functions formerly believed to be entirely involuntary, such as heart rate, blood pressure, and blood flow to various parts of the body. When you visualize certain changes that you'd like to take place in your body, they tend to occur – even though you may not fully understand, or be aware of, the underlying mechanisms. All that is needed is for you to visualize what you want to achieve. In this way you can, to some extent, help to bring it about.

Visualization may be considered a conscious programming of desired change through the use of positive images. Think of it as visual meditation, which is an important part of yoga practice (see Chapter 3, pages 41–2). Visualization enhances the effects of the physical exercises (*asanas*) and breathing exercises (*pranayama*) and helps promote a sense of calm, personal control, and confidence. These are invaluable to those experiencing the anxiety that not infrequently accompanies an asthma episode. Visualization can also be employed to reduce certain cravings, such as those for tobacco, a known asthma trigger.

Visualization need not be exclusively visual, however. As well as mental images, you can also create mental sounds, tastes, smells and sensations of textures and temperatures, thus enlisting the aid of all five senses – and of a sixth, also, which I call the 'S' sense. This I consider our 'essence', or the substance of all that we are.

Case Study
Before describing specific mental exercises, here is a story to illustrate how visualization can influence the course of an illness.

Six young male migraine sufferers aged between 10 and 13 were treated with various medicines, including pain relievers, with no success. They were then referred to psychologists, who tried to teach them a technique to raise the temperature of their hands. This hand-warming technique works on the principle that during times of anxiety and stress, blood flow to the hands is restricted. With relaxation, the hands become warm – and any congestion in the head, which contributes to the migraine, is relieved.

The boys in this study were overachievers, and so found it difficult to relax with this technique. They regarded the hand-warming as yet another exercise in which to attain excellence, and talked about scoring 90 or 100 percent. They were trying too hard, and therefore generating additional tension.

Now, almost desperate, the psychologists remembered earlier advice to make biofeedback imagery interesting to children. And so they invoked the image of the

Jedi Master Obi-Wan Kenobi, a character in the Star Wars movies. It was he who had taught Luke Skywalker to use 'The Force'.

The youngsters, who were familiar with the movies and with Kenobi's exhortations to relax and use inner strength to achieve goals, had no difficulty in visualizing the pertinent scenes, with coaching from their therapists. Actual dialogue from the movies, along with appropriate suggestions, were employed, for example: 'Remember, a Jedi can feel The Force flowing through him.'

Within three weeks, five of the young migraine sufferers were expert at hand-warming and could relax at will. Their migraines had disappeared. The other youngster took six weeks to attain the same goal. In follow-up examinations over a two-year period, the boys reported no further headaches.

The psychologists' conclusions about why 'The Force' worked so effectively in these cases are equally applicable to several other approaches used to stimulate self-healing and self-regulating powers. First, treatment is most successful when it increases an individual's sense of self-control, adequacy or self-mastery. Second, treatment is most effective when the person has implicit faith in the therapist and indeed in the treatment. Third, a pleasant, restful image on which to focus for a while is very therapeutic for the whole system. It fosters a state of relaxation, which enhances the power of our own inner self-repairing forces.

VISUALIZATION EXERCISES

An Exercise for Your Six Senses
This is an exercise in awareness. It will help put you in touch with the deep inner part of your being, something that tends to be neglected in the hustle and bustle of today's hectic way of life. It will also enable you to be more conscious of your surroundings and of your relationship with things around you. Do modify the instructions to suit your own special situation.

1   Sit comfortably with your spine well supported. Make a quick mental check of your body, from head to toe, and relax any particularly tense parts, such as your jaw and hands.

2   Feel a gentle breeze caressing your face, arms and legs. Sense its delicious coolness.

3   Picture a distant mountain range, tall and majestic, silhouetted against the sky.

4   Delight in the tantalizing smell of freshly-squeezed lemons which now claims your attention. Reach for the tall glass of lemonade beside you, and take a deep, refreshing drink. Savor the taste.

5   Hear the wind sighing in the evergreens; the leaves of the cherry trees rustling, and the sea-plane droning as it takes off from the river in the distance.

6   Now merge with your environment, until you begin to feel no separation from it. Feel a kinship with it. Imagine the trees to be your brothers and sisters, and the earth your mother. Think of the sky as your grandfather, and the moon as your grandmother. And the plane in its flight as your father, soaring towards the heavens like a mighty eagle. Then feel no fear or isolation. Only a sense of peace.

Notes
Create your own exercise for the six senses, based on your unique experiences, and compatible with your own belief system. Suggested settings include:

- a mountainside retreat
- a quiet lakeside setting
- a deserted beach
- a Japanese garden.

The ABC Exercise
Here's a visualization exercise to help you whenever you're having difficulty breathing, such as during an asthma flare-up. It consists of a mnemonic (memory aid) along with imagery and conscious breathing. I've chosen the mnemonic 'ABC', since most English-speaking people, children in particular, will find it easy to remember. You can, however, create your own memory aid.

1. At the onset of the episode, think ABC: A is for airways, B is for breathing, and C is for calm control. This will remind you of the sequence of steps to follow.

2. Willfully slow down your rate of breathing, as much as you possibly can. Unclench your teeth but keep your lips together, though not compressed. Breathe in through your nose, but pretend to breathe through your mouth. This will relax your throat and you will feel as though you're taking in more air than you otherwise would. If you have difficulty taking in one steady breath, divide the inhalation into small equal parts, as in the Sniffing Breath (see page 119).

3. As you breathe, imagine narrowed air passages widening as they let go of their tightness, thus allowing more oxygen to enter your lungs.

4. Breathe out as slowly as you can, through your nose or through pursed lips, as if cooling a hot drink, again visualizing a progressive relaxation of your airways. With each subsequent breath, mentally see the airways becoming wider and wider.

5. Repeat this process (steps 2 to 4) until you sense that you are calmer and your breathing is easier.

Notes

Use any imagery with which you can easily relate. For example, in steps 3 and 4, you may picture your narrowed air passages as small rubber tubes with kinks in them, and each breath you take slackening the kinks until they disappear altogether. Or you may, with your mind's eye, see tightened bands around your airways (small muscles around the bronchi and larger bronchioles) gradually relaxing with each respiration, giving more diameter to these passages, and a better supply of oxygen reaching your lungs.

With experimentation and frequent practice when not in difficulty, you will find the imagery that works best for you, so that you will be prepared for any flare-up that may occur.

Please refer also to Chapter 5, page 128, for positions that ease breathlessness. You may find the last of these – a sort of tripod position – useful during an asthma episode.

Candle Concentration

A common misconception is that concentration generates tension and fatigue, and depletes energy. The fact is, however, that concentrating or focusing on a particular object promotes alertness, feelings of safety, and productivity.

The balancing postures in Chapter 4 (pages 104–11) are useful in training you in the art of 'one-pointing', or focusing, with the benefits mentioned above. The following exercise also offers similar advantages.

CAUTION: To ensure safety, please supervise any young children practicing this exercise.

1   Place a lighted candle at or slightly below eye level, on a table, stool or other suitable prop.
2   Sit comfortably and observe good posture. Relax your jaw and breathe regularly throughout the exercise.
3   Look intently at the candle flame for a minute or two (Figure 122). Blink if you need to.
4   Now close your eyes and try to retain or recall the image of the flame. If it disappears, do not be anxious. Instead, mentally gaze in the direction of the flame and gently persuade it to come back.
5   After a minute or two, open your eyes. Relax.

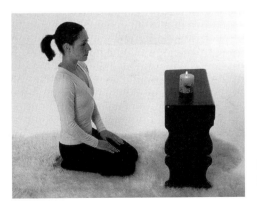

Fig. 122.
Candle Concentration

Each time you practice this technique, increase the length of time you spend looking at the flame, and that spent recalling its image.

Variation

Instead of a candle you may use any small, pleasing object, such as a fruit, a drawn design, or even a stone.

Coping with Anxiety and Panic

Part of yoga training is the practice of concentration, meditation and relaxation techniques. These help divert attention away from disturbing environmental stimuli. They also help you learn how to become calmer and more focused, and so gain a feeling of personal control and confidence. They give you a sense of empowerment so that you do not see yourself as wholly at the mercy of outside forces. Knowing that you have a measure of control over your body and your life is both comforting and invaluable, especially when facing or experiencing an asthma episode (also referred to as an asthma attack or flare-up). It helps, in addition, to counteract the anxiety that often accompanies such an episode. It combats the uncertainty and hopelessness that are associated with anxiety and prevents it from developing into panic (see Chapter 3, page 36).

What Is Anxiety?

Anxiety may be described as a vague, uncomfortable feeling of apprehension, dread, or danger from an unknown source. Psychologists have pointed out how it differs from fear. They say that the latter appears to be a relatively concrete state in which an immediate and identifiable danger is present, whereas the former tends to be more symbolic and less imminent – what psychologists call 'free-floating'.

Features of Anxiety

The key features of anxiety seem to be that it:

- is anticipatory – that is, it pertains to something perceived as harmful in the future; not necessarily physically harmful, but rather psychologically so, representing a threat to one's identity or being
- concerns symbolic dangers, generating what existential psychologists refer to as existential anxiety, or the loss of self
- involves dangers and adjustments of a highly ambiguous nature: the person experiencing the anxiety does not appear to have clear knowledge of what the danger is, when and how it will happen, or how it might be dealt with.

To the extent that its origins are unclear to the person experiencing it, anxiety generates the highly stressful feeling of uncertainty, and sometimes also one of helplessness.

Types of Anxiety

Ranging from mild to severe, anxiety presents itself in a number of forms and in various intensities: For some people it may be a short acute episode, while for others it may occur almost constantly. Health care professionals describe several types of anxiety, including:

- acute situational anxiety
- adjustment disorder
- generalized anxiety disorder
- panic disorder
- post-traumatic stress disorder
- phobias
- obsessive-compulsive disorder.

Common Signs and Symptoms of Anxiety

Some common symptoms include:

- a feeling of foreboding, that something harmful is about to happen
- dry mouth, difficulty swallowing, hoarseness
- unsteadiness of the hands, trembling
- muscle tension
- headaches
- sweating
- nausea, diarrhea (and accompanying weight loss)
- accelerated heart rate, palpitations, racing pulse
- rapid breathing, hyperventilation (see page 143)
- dizziness, feeling faint
- sleeplessness, nightmares
- irritability
- low energy, fatigue
- difficulty concentrating and/or remembering
- sexual impotence.

These signs and symptoms are a result of the activation of the body's 'fight or flight' response, in which there is an excess of the hormone adrenaline and of the catecholamines (hormones that act on nerve cells).

Aggravating Factors

The risk of anxiety increases with:

- stress from any source
- a family history of nervous disorders
- fatigue or overwork

- a medical illness
- lack of social supports.

Prevention

The first effective step toward controlling anxiety is to explore its possible causes. For this, it may be necessary to enlist the help of a health care professional. Once the probable source of anxiety has been identified, a plan can be devised to help you cope with it. This may involve lifestyle changes or medicines or both, and will probably include some form of daily relaxation (see Chapter 8).

Left untreated, anxiety may develop into more serious conditions such as panic attacks, phobias, or compulsive behaviors. It may even precipitate heart arrhythmia (irregular rhythm).

Treatment

Following laboratory studies to rule out any medical condition that may be producing anxiety, such as hyperthyroidism (overactive thyroid gland), any number of treatments may be instituted. These include:

- therapy to help you understand the specific (though unconscious) source or sources of the perceived threat
- learning and practicing techniques such as relaxation exercises (see Chapter 8), breathing exercises (Chapter 5), visualization exercises (Chapter 6), meditation and biofeedback, to help reduce muscle tension. Muscle tension is related to anxiety, and so if tense muscles can be made to relax, then anxiety will be reduced
- a regular exercise program to promote body–mind fitness. Please refer to Chapter 4 for the benefits you can expect to derive from yoga practice to better equip you for keeping your asthma under control. In this chapter you will also find exercise

precautions to take as necessary

- anti-anxiety or antidepressant medicines for short-term use (these are useful, for example, while adjustments to lifestyle are being made)
- sedative/hypnotic agents for the short-term treatment of sleep disturbances.

EIGHT HELPFUL HINTS

1. When you sense the beginnings of anxiety or you feel it increasing, stop and take a few slow, smooth breaths. Mentally tell yourself: 'This too will pass,' or a similar affirmation.
2. Learn to be assertive: to say 'no' when necessary.
3. Learn to express yourself. How can others know how you feel unless you tell them?
4. Learn to be decisive. Do not be afraid of making a well-thought-out decision. Stick to your decision once you have made it. (There is, however, room for reconsideration, in some cases.)
5. Concentrate on today. Yesterday is over, and what happens tomorrow depends on how you manage today.
6. Nurture yourself. This is not at all selfish; it is intelligent. The fitter you are, the better you can cope with various forms of stress.
7. Eat enough wholesome foods (see Chapter 9). Good nutrition is imperative for optimum body–mind wellness.
8. If your doctor has prescribed medicine to help you cope with anxiety and related states, be aware that it is usually a short-term expedient. Do not regard it as a substitute for using your own personal resources. Be sure you are knowledgeable about the medicine, its mode of action, and its side-effects. Discuss these issues with your doctor.

Hyperventilation

Of course, asthma sufferers will know that feelings of anxiety can also precede or accompany an asthma episode. Most of us tend to quicken our breathing in response to stress. Breathing may become so rapid that a state of hyperventilation (over-breathing) occurs.

Continued rapid breathing results in an oxygen surplus and carbon dioxide depletion. It is the carbon dioxide level in the body that determines the control of respiration in the brain.

If hyperventilation is prolonged, the extra oxygen constricts blood vessels and hinders the release of oxygen from the hemoglobin. Consequently, less blood will be carrying less oxygen to the body's tissues.

Hyperventilation leads to anxiety, which is commonly seen when asthma episodes occur. The person experiencing the episode often feels helpless and in the grip of something he or she is powerless to control, unless prepared to deal with it. The various yoga breathing, visualization, and relaxation exercises described in this book are excellent preparation for such occurrences.

Hyperventilation can also contribute to a fall in blood pressure, a feeling of lightheadedness, dizziness, nausea, and tingling or numbness of the hands and feet, and this could progress to cramps or other muscle spasms.

Should hyperventilation occur, you can try:

- slowing down your breathing, especially exhalation
- closing one nostril (with a thumb or fingers) and breathing slowly through the other (see also Alternate Nostril Breathing, page 120).

The following exercises will help you prevent anxiety and avert panic. They involve the use of your breath (a 'tool' you have with you wherever you are), which is closely linked to your emotions and emotional state. As such, practicing yoga breathing exercises will also help you control or avert an anxiety attack, as well, of course, as ameliorating asthma episodes.

The Whispering Breath

This exercise makes use of a technique called pursed-lip breathing. It allows the airways to remain open longer and reduces the amount of trapped air in the alveoli. It also allows a greater than usual volume of air to be exhaled. By prolonging exhalation, pursed-lip breathing promotes a sense of control: it trains you to control the rate and depth of your breathing. It therefore alleviates dyspnea (difficulty breathing) and the sense of anxiety or panic that not infrequently accompany it.

The Whispering Breath also helps improve concentration and promote general relaxation.

CAUTION: For safety, children using a lighted candle should be supervised.

1. Place a lighted candle on a prop in front of you, so that it is at eye level or slightly below. Sit comfortably and relax your body, particularly your jaw and facial muscles. Breathe regularly.
2. Inhale through your nose slowly, smoothly, and as deeply as you can without strain.
3. Through pursed lips, as if whistling or cooling a hot drink, blow at the candle flame. Do so slowly, smoothly, gently and with control. The object is to make the flame flicker, but not to put it out (Figure 123).
4. At the end of your exhalation, close your mouth but do not compress your lips or clench your teeth.
5. Repeat steps 2 to 4 as many times as you wish, in smooth succession.
6. Resume regular breathing.

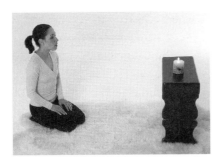

Fig. 123.
The Whispering Breath

Notes

Once you have mastered this exercise, you can dispense with the candle. Close your eyes and blow at an imaginary flame.

Try practicing The Whispering Breath while lying down, standing, or walking up or down the stairs. Keep your eyes open and hold on to the handrail for safety.

Anti-Anxiety Breath

I call this exercise a non-pharmaceutical anxiolytic (an agent, such as a medicine, used to diminish or counteract anxiety). As its name suggests, it is useful for counteracting anxiety and averting panic. It is also effective in managing troubling emotions such as apprehension, frustration, and anger.

When you slow down your respirations, it is virtually impossible to panic. The Anti-Anxiety Breath trains you in lengthening your exhalation, which many people with asthma find difficult.

1   Sit upright and observe good posture. Close your eyes or keep them open, whichever you prefer. Relax your jaw. (You may also practice this exercise while lying down or standing.)
2   Inhale quietly through your nose as slowly, smoothly, and deeply as you can, without strain.
3   Exhale through your nose as slowly, smoothly, and completely as you can without force.
4   Before inhaling again, do a slow mental count: 'one thousand', 'two thousand'. (This prolongs exhalation and prevents hyperventilation.)
5   Repeat steps 2 to 4 again and again, in smooth succession, until your breathing rate has become slower, and you feel calm.
6   Resume regular breathing.

Notes

- If you wish, you can combine imagery with this exercise. Visualize filling your body with positive qualities such as courage, patience, and hope as you inhale. As you exhale, imagine sending away, with the outgoing breath, negative influences such as fear, gloom, and disappointment.
- Instead of exhaling through your nose, you may do so through pursed lips, as in The Whispering Breath (see page 145).
- Other practices to help condition you in extending your exhalation include: blowing a balloon; blowing bubbles; singing or chanting; playing a wind instrument such as a recorder, flute, or clarinet.

The Feelings Breath

The ancient practitioners of yoga were probably the first to discover the close relationship between breathing and the emotions. This link has now been substantiated, and today breathing is commonly used as a therapeutic tool to help reduce stress and bring about a state of calm and self-control.

Changes in feelings, especially if they are intense, are reflected in patterns of breathing, affecting the smooth continuous flow of the breath. Fear, for example, produces fast, shallow breathing. Anger results in short, quick inhalations and strong, rapid exhalations, and in anxiety states, which are frequently seen during asthma episodes, breathing is also fast and sometimes irregular, thus compounding the difficulty. Feelings such as joy, love and forgiveness induce slow, smooth, even respirations by contrast, and a sense of peace and wellbeing.

Because the relationship between breathing and our feelings is reciprocal, however, we can create a change in our emotional climate by consciously altering our pattern of breathing. (Our respiratory system is the only bodily system that is both voluntary and involuntary.)

Working with the breath, in fact, can be one of the quickest ways of overcoming painful or otherwise difficult emotions.

Coping with Anxiety
and Panic

1 Sit or lie with your spine in good alignment and supported if necessary, for maximum comfort. Relax your jaw, throat, and facial muscles. Relax your shoulders, chest, abdomen, back, and hands. Close your eyes and breathe regularly through your nose.

2 Shift your focus of attention to that part of your body where you feel the difficult emotion most (your abdomen, chest, neck, or small of the back, for example). Breathe into it, as it were. Breathe in through your nose slowly, smoothly, and as deeply as you can without strain.

3 Now breathe out slowly, smoothly and completely, without force. Maintain an awareness of the emotion as you breathe: Do not try to suppress it. Feel and experience it without fear.

4 Repeat steps 2 and 3 as many times as you wish.

5 Take a few deep, diaphragmatic breaths (see pages 115–17).

6 Again, focus your attention on that part of your body where you feel the emotion most. Breathe into it with a slow, smooth, comfortably deep inhalation.

7 As you exhale slowly and steadily, visualize the emotion (sadness, resentment, frustration or fear, for instance) dissolving with the outgoing breath.

8 Repeat steps 6 and 7 as many times as you wish, or until you sense a lessening in the intensity of the emotion.

9 Take a few deep diaphragmatic breaths.

10 Now think of a pleasant emotion (such as a feeling of goodwill, affection or forgiveness). Try to locate the part of your body where you feel it most.

11 Breathe into that area through your nose, with a slow, smooth, comfortably deep inhalation.

12 As you breathe out slowly, smoothly and completely, without force, visualize sending this warm feeling toward the person or persons you had originally perceived as the source of your difficult emotion, or toward someone you wish to receive this benevolent sentiment.

13 Repeat steps 10 to 12 as many times as you wish, or until you experience a sense of relief or peace.

14 Finish the exercise with a few deep diaphragmatic breaths. Open your eyes. Do a few leisurely body stretches, if you wish, before resuming your usual activities. Breathe regularly.

Note
Other exercises to try when dealing with troublesome feelings are: Alternate Nostril
Breathing and the Sniffing Breath (described in Chapter 5, pages 120 and 119) and
the Anti-Anxiety Breath described earlier in this chapter (page 146).

Relaxation Exercises

Apart from poor posture, perhaps nothing affects efficient breathing as much as tension buildup. Accumulated tension inhibits the free movement of the chest wall and the abdomen, thus restricting the movement of important respiratory structures such as the diaphragm. Complete muscular relaxation, by contrast, reduces oxygen consumption and carbon dioxide production. It also helps lessen the intensity of states such as over-excitement and anxiety, which not infrequently accompany asthma episodes.

Increasing evidence supports the efficacy of relaxation techniques in counteracting high levels of muscular tension, which detract from efficient respiration. This chapter, therefore, offers a number of such techniques to help you eliminate tension from your whole body (systemic relaxation), in a progressive manner. It also offers suggestions for preventing tension buildup in individual areas (local relaxation), such as the neck and shoulders.

Local Relaxation

Some of the warm-up exercises in Chapter 4 can also be practiced to prevent tension from building up in respiratory muscles and other structures. These include the Figure-Eight (page 47) and Shoulder Rotation (page 48). The Posture Clasp (page 65) and the Chest Expander (page 66) are excellent for relaxing the chest and upper back muscles, while the Dog Stretch (page 98) is superb for reducing accumulated tension in the legs and feet. The Lion, described later in this chapter (page 158), is wonderful for eliminating tightness from the face and throat.

Systemic Relaxation

The Rag Doll (page 61), the Curling Leaf (page 78), the Half Shoulderstand (page 100), and the Full Shoulderstand (page 101) are just four of the many techniques described in this book that are effective for relaxing the whole body.

Virtually all the breathing exercises in Chapter 5 are useful for releasing accumulated tension and promoting general relaxation, particularly Rhythmic Diaphragmatic Breathing (pages 115–17), Alternate Nostril Breathing (pages 120–2), The Whispering Breath (pages 145–6), the Anti-Anxiety Breath (page 146), and the Feelings Breath (page 147).

In addition, the following two postures are worthy of consideration and practice to counteract tension that has gathered insidiously in the body, and to induce all-over relaxation.

Stick Posture

1 Lie on a mat with your legs stretched out in front and your arms at your sides. Breathe regularly.

2 Inhale slowly, smoothly, and as deeply as you comfortably can as you bring your arms overhead. If possible, place the palms of your hands together. At the same time, stretch your legs to their fullest comfortable extent, pulling your toes towards you and pushing your heels away (Figure 124). The entire stretch should be done in one smooth, conscious movement in synchronization with a slow inhalation.

3 Maintain this all-body stretch for a few seconds, but do not hold your breath.

4 Release the stretch as you exhale, and bring your arms back at your sides. Rest.

5 You may repeat the exercise once. Rest afterwards.

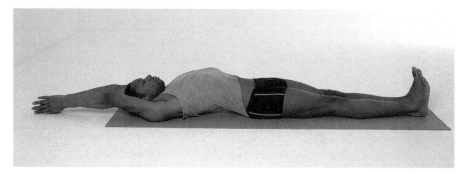

Fig. 124.
Stick Posture (lying down)

Variation: Stick Posture

You may also practice the Stick Posture while standing, modifying the instructions above accordingly.

The Crocodile

1 Lie on your abdomen with your legs stretched out and comfortably separated. (You may place a thin pillow or cushion under your hips.)

2 Fold your arms and rest your head on them, with your head turned to the side. Close your eyes (Figure 125). Breathe regularly throughout the exercise.

3 Mentally go over your body, concentrating on one part at a time, giving each part a silent suggestion to let go of tension and to relax completely. Include: the feet, legs, hips, upper back, abdomen, chest, arms and hands, neck, head and facial muscles.

4 If your thoughts stray, gently guide them back and continue the exercise.

5 Finish the exercise with several minutes of slow, rhythmical breathing, allowing your body to sink more fully into your mat with each exhalation.

6 Roll onto your side, and use your hands to help you into a sitting position.

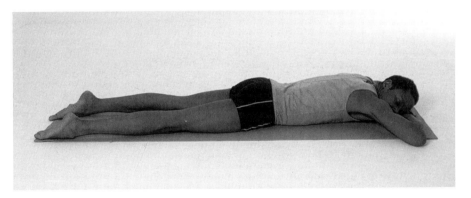

Fig. 125.
The Crocodile

Pose of Tranquility (Savasana)

Perhaps the most wonderful of all relaxation techniques, one loved by millions of yoga practitioners all over the world, is the Pose of Tranquility, or *Savasana*.

This exercise in the art of deep relaxation helps break the fear–tension–pain cycle, thus making it easier to cope with distress. It has been used with admirable success in a number of areas including: childbirth, competitive sports, to help lower high blood pressure, and in the treatment of anxiety states and phobias.

Deep relaxation brings to the surface muscular and nervous tensions, the existence of which you may not have been aware. You can then release them voluntarily. In doing so, you contribute to a restoration of the natural harmony between body and mind, which characterizes integrity and good health.

When you habitually practice deep relaxation, beneficial changes occur in the functioning of all the body's systems, not only during practice, but also long afterwards. Some of these changes include:

- a calmer mental state
- better emotional balance
- a more even temper; more control
- improved concentration
- better productivity
- blood pressure lowered to within normal limits.

1   Lie on your back with your legs stretched out in front of you. Separate your feet to discourage a buildup of tension in your legs. Move your arms away from your sides to prevent an accumulation of tension in your shoulders. Keep your arms straight but relaxed, and the palms of your hands upturned. Close your eyes. Unclench your teeth to relax your jaw, but keep your mouth closed without compressing your lips. Breathe regularly (Figure 126).

2   Focus your attention on your feet. Pull your toes towards you, pushing your heels away. Hold the ankle position briefly but do not hold your breath. Now relax your feet and ankles.

3   Stiffen your legs, locking your knee joints. Hold briefly. Relax your knees.

4   Tighten your buttock muscles. Hold the tightness for a few seconds. Release the tightness.

5   On an exhalation, press the small of your back (waist level) towards or against the mat. Hold the pressure as long as your exhalation lasts, then release the pressure as you inhale. Keep breathing regularly.

6   Inhale and squeeze your shoulderblades together. Hold the squeeze as long as your inhalation lasts. Release the squeeze as you exhale. Continue breathing regularly.

7   On an exhalation, tighten your abdominal muscles. Hold the tightness as long as the exhalation lasts. Inhale and relax. Breathe regularly.

8   Take a slow, smooth, deep inhalation without strain, imagining that you are filling the top, middle, and bottom of your lungs. Be aware of your chest expanding and your abdomen rising. Exhale slowly, smoothly and steadily, imagining that you are emptying your lungs by degrees. Be aware of your chest and abdomen relaxing. Continue breathing regularly.

9   Tighten your hands into fists, straighten your arms and raise them off the mat. Hold the stiffness briefly, then let the arms and hands fall to the mat, free of stiffness. Relax them.

10 Keep your arms relaxed, but shrug your shoulders as if to touch your ears with them. Hold the shrug briefly, then relax your shoulders.

11 Gently roll your head from side to side a few times. Reposition your head and keep breathing regularly.

12 Exhaling, open your eyes and mouth widely; stick your tongue out; tense all your facial muscles. Inhale and close your mouth and eyes and relax your facial muscles. Breathe regularly.

13 Lie relaxed for as many minutes as you can spare. Give your body weight up to the surface that supports it. Each time you exhale, let your body sink more deeply into that surface, increasingly relaxed.

14 Before getting up, rotate your ankles, roll your head gently from side to side and leisurely stretch your limbs. Never get up suddenly. Rather, do so slowly and carefully.

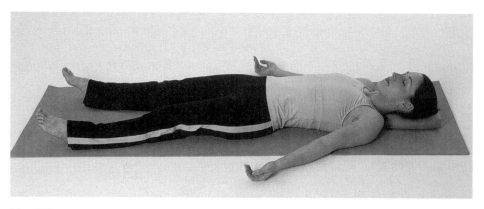

Fig. 126.
Pose of Tranquility

Notes

- If you are unwell, you may practice the Pose of Tranquility in bed or in an easy chair. Modify the exercise instructions accordingly.
- You may practice it lying on your back, with your knees bent and your lower legs (not your calves) resting on a padded chair seat or sofa.
- Use whatever props you need to support your body, particularly your neck and lower back, so that you are absolutely comfortable. Suitable aids include folded towels, folded blankets, cushions and pillows.
- Keep a sweater or blanket and a pair of warm socks nearby. Use them to prevent you from becoming cold as your body cools down during relaxation.
- In step 13 of the instructions, use imagery with which you are comfortable. You may, for example, visualize yourself lying on a warm, sandy beach in summer, with a soft breeze caressing your face, hair and body, as you delight in pleasant memories.
- Practice the Pose of Tranquility any time you need to re-energize yourself, such as after a demanding day or a particularly trying experience that has left you feeling exhausted. Practice it when you feel anxious.
- Practice this technique in a quiet place where you won't be interrupted for at least 20 minutes.

- When you are well versed in the technique, you may dispense with alternately tightening and relaxing muscle groups and simply give mental suggestions to the various parts of your body to let go of tension and relax. For example, as you focus attention on your feet, you may mentally say to them: 'Feet, let go of your tightness; relax.' Work from the feet upwards, and remember to include the facial muscles.

- You may record the instructions for the Pose of Tranquility onto a tape-recorder (or ask a friend to do so). Speak slowly and soothingly. Listen to the recording as the need arises.

The Lion

Wonderful for helping rid your jaw and tongue of unneeded tension and so facilitate unrestricted breathing, the Lion is also useful in averting a sore throat or in reducing its intensity and duration.

1 Sit on your heels in The Firm Posture (see page 64). Breathe regularly.
2 Inhale slowly and smoothly.
3 As you exhale, open your mouth fully; stick out your tongue; open your eyes wide as if staring; tense the muscles of your face and throat. You may also stiffen your arms and fingers (Figures 127 and 128).
4 When your exhalation is complete, pull in your tongue, close your mouth without clenching your teeth, and relax your face and throat. Relax your arms and hands. Close your eyes and breathe regularly.
5 Rest briefly, visualizing all the built-up tension draining from your face, throat and tongue.
6 Repeat the exercise (steps 3 to 5) once. Repeat it later, if you wish.

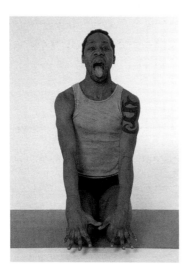

Fig. 127.
The Lion: Front view

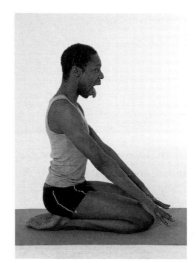

Fig. 128.
The Lion: Side view

Nutrition Matters

One of the roles of good nutrition is to strengthen the body and help you withstand unhealthy environmental influences, such as air pollution. Another is to increase your resistance to infections such as rhinitis and sinusitis, which are asthma triggers.

This chapter highlights certain essential nutrients considered of particular importance to asthma sufferers. It also brings to your attention certain foods and food additives, and their possible unpleasant effects. Do not, however, remove any food or food substance from your diet, and do not take any dietary supplements, without first consulting a trained professional such as a doctor or a nutritionist.

Food Allergies

Some foods can produce a number of unpleasant reactions in those who are sensitive to them. The most common of these are:

- eggs
- milk and other dairy products
- peanuts (which are classified as legumes)
- seeds such as sesame
- nuts
- fish

- shrimp and other shellfish
- soy products.

Some food additives and preservatives can also produce adverse reactions. These include sulfites, which are a food and beverage preservative used to retard spoilage and make foods fresh-looking. The names by which they are listed on labels are: sulfur dioxide, sodium sulfite, sodium and potassium bisulfite, and sodium and potassium metabisulfite. They have also been used as preservatives in medications, including some nebulizer solutions.

Tartrazine, which is a yellow dye, has also been added to foods such as margarine and also to some medicines, and has been known to trigger asthmatic episodes in sensitive individuals.

Food Intolerance

Some adverse reactions to certain foods are a result of food intolerance, rather than allergy. An example is lactose intolerance in people who lack the enzyme lactase, which is needed to digest milk sugar (lactose). Symptoms of lactose intolerance include abdominal pain, bloating, and diarrhea.

SYMPTOMS OF ADVERSE REACTIONS

The most common type of allergic reaction to eating certain foods is hives: red, itchy, swollen areas that erupt on the skin. Other manifestations of food allergy include:

- itching and swelling of the mouth
- irritation of the throat
- abdominal cramps, vomiting and diarrhea.

Food allergies can also induce an asthma episode in asthma sufferers.

In some cases, a food allergy can produce a severe reaction known as *anaphylaxis*. Symptoms include:

- difficulty breathing (dyspnea)
- violent cough
- chest constriction
- cyanosis of the skin (causing it to take on a bluish tinge) and mucous membranes
- skin eruptions
- rapid pulse.

This type of severe reaction can prove fatal if not treated promptly.

If you are at risk of having a severe allergic reaction to an allergen, you and your doctor should devise an emergency plan. In the case of a child, his or her teachers, school nurse and any child-minders or baby-sitters should be made aware of the allergy, and of the plan for managing the symptoms.

Your doctor may prescribe an epinephrine kit. When this medication is administered at the onset of severe symptoms, it can halt their progression. It is advisable to seek prompt medical attention even after an anaphylactic reaction has been brought under control, to prevent the reappearance of symptoms and to avert danger.

Eating for Protection

Current research indicates that a diet rich in certain nutrients can help the immune system function optimally, and so protect the body from infection. This is an important consideration for people with asthma.

NUTRIENTS TO HEAL AND PROTECT

Nutrition aims at maintaining good health and rebuilding it when it is impaired. It is essentially what we eat that supplies the raw material for building and repairing the body's various components. Nutrients from the diet are processed by the digestive system and transported to every cell, tissue, and organ.

When the body is under stress, as occurs for example in an infection, the demand for certain nutrients increases. As healing takes place, the body uses up nutrients at a faster rate than usual.

In this chapter I shall highlight nutrients that appear particularly beneficial to people with asthma. It is worth remembering, however, that all nutrients work together for the harmonious functioning of the entire system.

Antioxidants

Antioxidants are agents that prevent or inhibit oxidation, a process whereby a substance combines with oxygen and produces free radicals. These have been referred to as 'mischievous molecules' that damage cells. Antioxidants include: vitamins A, C and E, and the mineral selenium.

VITAMIN A

An anti-infection vitamin, this nutrient helps build resistance to respiratory and other infections. It is also useful for maintaining the health of mucous membranes, and the disease-fighting properties of tears, saliva, and sweat.

Food Sources
*   fresh vegetables, especially the intensely green and yellow/orange ones such as broccoli, carrots, parsley and sweet potatoes

- fresh fruit, particularly apricots, cantaloupe melons, mangoes, papaya and peaches
- milk and milk products
- fish liver oils.

VITAMIN C

Vitamin C has long been known to help reduce the severity of minor infections. It is a natural antihistamine (counteracting the action of histamine, a chemical substance released when tissues are injured). The runny nose and the swollen, inflamed lining of the nasal passages that accompany a cold, for instance, are due to the effects of histamine.

Vitamin C also has anti-stress properties, and it contributes to the body's utilization of oxygen and the maintenance of a healthy blood circulation.

Food Sources
- apricots, berries, cantaloupe melons, cherries, citrus fruits
- rosehips (the seed pods of wild roses)
- cabbage, green and red peppers
- mustard and cress.

Flavonoids
Associated with vitamin C are compounds known as flavonoids, which protect against free radical damage. They also have anti-inflammatory, anti-allergy and anti-viral properties.

One of the most powerful of the flavonoids is quercetin, which is also an antioxidant. In the diets of people studied worldwide, onions are the chief source of this flavonoid.

A diet rich in fresh fruits and vegetables is the best way to ensure an adequate daily intake of flavonoids. Try to include the following rich sources:

- apples
- cabbage
- cranberries
- garlic
- peppers.

VITAMIN E

One of the anti-stress nutrients, vitamin E improves circulation and helps alleviate fatigue. Along with vitamin C, it can protect the lungs against air pollution.

Food Sources
- Brussels sprouts
- eggs
- fresh fruits
- green leafy vegetables
- legumes
- nuts
- seeds
- unrefined vegetable oils
- wheat germ
- whole grains.

SELENIUM

Selenium is a trace mineral, needed in small amounts to maintain healthy circulation and to reinforce the body's immune system.

Food Sources
- apple cider vinegar
- asparagus
- brewer's yeast

- eggs
- garlic
- mushrooms
- seafood
- sesame seeds
- unrefined cereals
- wheat germ
- whole grains.

The B Vitamins

The B-vitamin complex consists of more than 20 vitamins, all working together. They help counteract the harmful effects of high stress levels, and they influence all components of the immune system. A deficiency in any one of the B vitamins can result in low energy. The harder you work and the less sleep you obtain, the greater is your need for the B vitamins.

Food Sources
- brewer's yeast
- green leafy vegetables
- legumes
- wheat germ
- whole grains and cereals.

VITAMIN B5 (PANTOTHENIC ACID)

This vitamin enhances immunity to disease and it also has antihistamine properties. In addition, it is useful in counteracting fatigue and boosting energy. Vitamin B5, moreover, is important for the normal functioning of adrenal gland secretions, which play a vital role in stress reactions.

Food Sources
- avocados
- brewer's yeast
- broccoli
- brown rice
- cabbage
- green vegetables
- legumes
- milk
- mushrooms
- sweet potatoes
- unrefined vegetable oils
- wheat germ
- whole grains.

VITAMIN B6 (PYRIDOXINE)

Vitamin B6 is very important for maintaining a healthy immune system. It also has an antihistamine action, and is an essential nutrient for the health of mucous membranes.

Food Sources
- apples
- bananas
- brewer's yeast
- brown rice
- buckwheat flour
- cantaloupe melons
- carrots
- green leafy vegetables
- tomatoes
- wheat germ
- whole grains.

VITAMIN B12

Essential for the production and regeneration of red blood cells, vitamin B12 is also important for the body's proper utilization of fats, carbohydrates, and protein. It may, in addition, have a regulating effect on the immune system.

Food Sources
- eggs
- milk products
- tempeh (a sort of cheese made from fermented soy beans).

Other Nutrients

ESSENTIAL FATTY ACIDS (EFAs)

EFAs consist of the omega-3 and the omega-6 fatty acids. They are called 'essential' because the body needs them. They are a necessary component of the fatty film that coats the skin's surface, a film that is important for protection against the entry of disease-causing organisms. EFAs, moreover, aid in weight reduction by burning saturated fats. Because the body cannot produce them, they must be obtained from food. An EFA deficiency could result in eczema, which is sometimes associated with allergy.

Food Sources
- the oils of certain seeds and nuts, such as flax, sunflower and sesame seeds, and those of the evening primrose plant
- wheat germ
- soy bean and peanut oils
- avocados
- most nuts (except Brazil and cashew nuts).

CALCIUM

In addition to its well-known role in maintaining the health of bones and teeth, calcium is needed for healthy nervous tissue, and is considered an anti-stress mineral. It can also help to combat sleeplessness. Calcium, moreover, is required to keep your heart beating regularly, and it helps to metabolize your body's iron.

Food Sources
- blackstrap molasses
- carob powder
- citrus fruits
- dried figs
- green vegetables
- milk
- peanuts
- sesame seeds
- soy beans
- sunflower seeds
- walnuts.

IRON

Iron is an essential part of immune system enzymes and proteins. It is a vital component of hemoglobin, which transports oxygen to all the body's cells.

Unless you are menstruating, have suffered significant blood-loss, or are clinically anemic, you should avoid taking iron supplements unless they have been prescribed by a doctor. Excess iron in the body can accumulate to toxic levels, and this can interfere with immunity.

Food Sources
- blackstrap molasses
- brewer's yeast

- Brussels sprouts
- cauliflower
- dried fruits
- egg yolk
- kiwi fruit
- leafy vegetables
- seaweed
- seeds
- Sharon fruit (persimmon)
- strawberries
- watermelon
- wheat germ
- whole grains.

MAGNESIUM

Magnesium is needed by every cell of the body, since it is essential for the synthesis of protein and the utilization of fats. Known as an anti-stress mineral, magnesium aids in combating depression. It also promotes the health of the cardiovascular system (heart and blood vessels). Symptoms of magnesium deficiency include: fatigue, weakness, nervous tension, and insomnia. Magnesium also appears to play an important role in a number of biochemical reactions that are important to lung function: it may enhance the strength of respiratory muscles, relax the smooth muscle of airways so as to facilitate dilatation (expansion) of the bronchioles, and reduce airway inflammation. Studies have shown that during an asthma episode, blood levels of magnesium are low while histamine levels are high.

Food Sources
- alfalfa sprouts
- almonds and other nuts eaten fresh from the shell
- apples
- beetroot tops
- blackstrap molasses

- brown rice
- celery
- chard
- citrus fruits
- green leafy vegetables
- peas
- potatoes
- sesame and sunflower seeds
- soy beans
- wheat bran
- wheat germ
- whole grains.

POTASSIUM

Working along with the mineral sodium, potassium helps maintain the electrical and chemical balance between tissue cells and blood. It is therefore crucial to the functioning of the lungs, heart, blood vessels, and nerves.

The two nutrients sodium and potassium must be in balance so as to maintain muscle contractions and the normal transmission of nerve signals.

Potassium also plays an important part in the release of energy from proteins, carbohydrates, and fats. It can, in addition, contribute to clear thinking by facilitating the supply of oxygen to the brain. It may also enhance allergy treatment.

Potassium helps maintain the body's acid–base and fluid balance, which directly affect breathing. (Acid–base balance refers to the mechanisms by which the acidity and alkalinity of body fluids are kept in a state of equilibrium.)

Food Sources
- bananas
- wholegrain cereals
- citrus fruits
- green leafy vegetables
- legumes
- mint leaves
- nuts
- potatoes
- watercress
- watermelon.

ZINC

Zinc is an anti-viral agent and a vital component of the immune system. It is essential for the proper functioning of more than 70 enzyme systems in the body. A zinc deficiency is linked to several health disorders, including a lowered resistance to infection.

Food Sources
- brewer's yeast
- cheese
- eggs
- lima (butter) beans
- green beans
- mushrooms
- non-fat dry milk
- nuts
- pumpkin seeds
- soy beans
- sunflower seeds
- wheat germ
- whole grains.

Water

Although it is not generally thought of as a nutrient, water is nevertheless the most important substance we consume. It is the principal constituent of body fluids, and also the medium in which nutrients are transported to all cells and wastes removed.

Water helps prevent dehydration and combat some infections. Absence of moisture, for even a few minutes, can destroy the delicate cilia (see page 5) which help to rid the respiratory system of debris.

The surface of the lungs must be moistened with water to facilitate the uptake of oxygen and the excretion of carbon dioxide. Water, therefore, enhances oxygen intake into the bloodstream. Water, in addition, thins mucus to allow it to drain more easily.

All liquids provide water, but the best sources include: unsweetened juices, non-caffeinated drinks such as herbal teas and milk, and mineral water. (Remember to check with your doctor or nutritionist regarding your use of herbal remedies, even in tea form.)

Weight Control

Excess weight has been linked to a number of health disorders, including high blood pressure, diabetes, and coronary artery disease. In the case of people with asthma, where the respiratory system is already stressed, added body weight makes breathing more difficult, particularly if it increases abdominal mass. This restricts free diaphragmatic movement so that breathing becomes difficult: the diaphragm has to push against a heavy abdomen.

Nutrient Antagonists

Agents that counteract the health-promoting properties of the vitamins, minerals, and other nutrients in the food and drink we consume are known as *antagonists*.

The following are among the most notable nutrient antagonists:

- the regular intake of acetylsalicylic acid (aspirin), which increases the requirement for vitamin C
- oral contraceptive pills, which act against the B vitamins and zinc
- rancid oils and other rancid foods, which destroy vitamin E
- some commercial laxatives, especially mineral oil, which can contribute to a deficiency of the B vitamins and vitamin C
- smoking, which destroys the B vitamins and vitamin C, and which also reduces vital oxygen supplies. Smoking also damages the cilia (see page 5)
- high alcohol intake, which is antagonistic to several essential vitamins and minerals. Alcohol also causes weight gain without providing useful nutrients
- too much caffeine (as in coffee and some soft drinks), which adversely affects the circulatory and respiratory systems
- high-protein diets, which may contribute to the excretion of essential nutrients such as calcium
- lack of exercise, which impairs delivery of vital nutrients to body tissues.

A Nutrition Checklist

- Reduce your intake of high-fat foods, which contribute to heart and blood-vessel diseases and to weight gain.
- Avoid high-protein diets, which place extra demands on the body and which can increase the need for other nutrients such as the B vitamins.
- Ensure a regular intake of dietary fiber (roughage), as found in fresh fruits, vegetables and whole grains, to prevent disorders such as constipation, and to help attain and maintain a trim, healthy body.

- Avoid using over-processed foods (including many convenience foods), which often contain additives and preservatives, and which are frequently devoid of important nutrients.
- Reduce sodium (salt) added to food during preparation and cooking, or at the table. High sodium intake has been linked to high blood pressure.
- Cut down on consumption of refined sugars, which have been implicated in conditions such as obesity and diabetes.
- Decrease or eliminate caffeine intake. Instead, drink beverages such as water, unsweetened juices, herbal teas and milk.
- Avoid substances known to be antagonistic to essential nutrients, such as alcohol, tobacco smoke, and commercial laxatives.
- If you are troubled by symptoms of hypoglycemia (low blood sugar), replace your usual three large meals with five or six smaller, nutritious ones, spaced evenly throughout the day, to help maintain adequate bloodsugar levels.
- Be knowledgeable and aware of any foods of which you are intolerant, or to which you are allergic. Follow the directions of your doctor or nutritionist regarding this.
- When shopping for food and beverages, read labels carefully, alert for the presence of any ingredients that may trigger asthma symptoms.
- Store, prepare and cook food in ways that conserve nutrients.
- Try to make mealtimes unhurried and pleasant. Chew food properly and do not overeat. An overloaded stomach can impede unrestricted breathing.
- Consult your doctor or nutritionist before taking any medication or supplement. Some of these can interact unfavorably with each other or with certain foods and drinks.

Looking Forward

Asthma is considered to be well controlled when it doesn't wake you up at night, when symptoms are absent, when you need bronchodilators for short-term relief only minimally, and when you can carry out your usual activities without bothersome side effects from asthma medicines. Taking certain preventive measures and complying with treatments prescribed by your doctor (see Chapter 2) can help you achieve satisfactory asthma control and enable you to live a joyous and productive life.

Experts agree that self-management is a key component in the successful control of asthma. Self-management includes a thorough understanding of the condition through accurate, up-to-date information; taking the precautions mentioned above; and responsible use of prescribed medications and your active involvement in treatment, as opposed to being only a passive recipient of treatment. It also includes the ability to draw upon your inner resources, to complement outer resources such as those provided by health-care professionals.

In technologically advanced societies, people tend to be impressed by and gravitate towards the visible, tangible things that are often also complex and costly. They tend to dismiss as insignificant those small, sometimes intangible things that are uncomplicated and inexpensive, such as the rich personal resources that they have with and within them: their muscles, their powers of concentration, and their ability to form mental pictures (visualize), to give only a few examples. And yet, small things are often vital, essential components of larger ones.

Crucial to effective self-management is your ability to draw upon those natural resources you have with and within you, and which are with you no matter where you are: your body, your mind and your breath.

Yoga practices train you to do this. They help you to gain an awareness of those inner 'tools' and to use them to full advantage, not only when you are experiencing difficulties, but also in your everyday activities, to cope with life's inevitable ups and downs. They thus help you to gain a measure of control over your life and to feel that you are not entirely at the mercy of outside forces. They consequently foster a wonderful sense of empowerment. Many world-class athletes with asthma are cognizant of these facts. They refuse to allow asthma to stop them from doing what they want to do in life. They choose what they want to do. They do not permit the disorder to dictate what they should do. They can do this because they take good care of their asthma and keep it under control. You can, too.

Resource Organizations

The following organizations provide information which people with asthma, or who have a relative with asthma, will find useful.

USA

American Lung Association
61 Broadway, 6th Floor
New York, NY 10006
(212) 315-8700

Allergy and Asthma Network/Mothers of Asthmatics, Inc.
3554 Chain Bridge Road, Suite 200
Fairfax, VA 22030
(703) 385-4403

Asthma and Allergy Foundation of America
1233 20th Street NW, Suite 402
Washington, DC 20036
(202) 466-7643

National Jewish Medical and Research Center
1400 Jackson Street
Denver, CO 80206
1-800-222-LUNG (5864)
outside the USA: (303) 388-4461/7700
lungline@njc.org

American Academy of Allergy, Asthma & Immunology
611 Wells Street
Milwaukee, WI 53202
(414) 272-6071
info@aaaai.org

CANADA

Allergy/Asthma Information Association National Office
130 Bridgeland Avenue, Suite 424
Toronto, ON M6A 1Z4
(416) 783 8944

The Lung Association National Office
3 Raymond Street, Suite 300
Ottawa ON K1R 1A3
(613) 569 6411
info@lung.ca

British Columbia Lung Association
2675 Oak Street
Vancouver, BC V6H 2K2
1-800 665 5864

UK

The British Lung Foundation
78 Hatton Garden
London EC1N 8LD
020 7831 5831
info@britishlungfoundation.com

Asthma Research Council
12 Pembridge Square
London W2 4EH

British Thoracic Society
17 Doughty Street
London WC1N 2PL
020 7831 8778

Yoga Therapy Centre
Homeopathic Hospital
60 Great Ormond Street
London WC1N 3HR
020 7419 7911 (Thursdays & Fridays)
www.yogatherapy.org

Respiratory Support and Sleep Centre
Papworth Hospital
Cambridge
Cambs CB3 8RE
01480 830541

UK College for Complementary Healthcare Studies
St Charles Hospital
Exmoor Street
London W10 6DZ
020 8964 1206

AUSTRALIA

National Asthma Campaign
5th Floor, 615 St Kilda Road
Melbourne, Victoria 3004
1800 032495

The Thoracic Society of Australia and New Zealand
145 Macquarie Street
Sydney NSW 2000
61 2 9256 5457
admin@thoracic.org.au

Glossary

Accessory breathing muscles   Muscles in the neck, shoulders, chest and back which help the main respiratory muscles during strenuous exercise, and when breathing becomes difficult

Adrenal glands   Two small triangular-shaped endocrine glands, one above each kidney

Adrenaline   Hormone secreted by the medullae (central portions) of the adrenal glands

Adverse effects   Undesirable effects

Allergen   Any substance that can induce allergy

Allergy   Condition in which the body has an immune reaction to a substance that is normally harmless

Alveolus   Air sac in the lung (plural: alveoli)

Anaphylaxis   An allergic hypersensitivity reaction of the body to a foreign protein or drug

Anemia   Deficiency in either the quality or quantity of red blood cells

Angina   Usually refers to angina pectoris, which is severe pain and constriction about the heart

Antibody   A protein produced by certain cells in response to a specific antigen. Also called immunoglobulin, or Ig

Antihistamine   Any agent that counteracts the effect of histamine

Anti-inflammatory agent   Medicine that counteracts inflammation

Antioxidant   An agent that prevents or inhibits oxidation

Asana   A yoga physical exercise; a posture comfortably held

Beta-agonists   A class of quick-relief medicine which causes relaxation of smooth muscle, and dilatation (widening) of airways. Also known as beta adrenergic receptor agonists

Bronchi   Branches of the respiratory passageway; the two main branches leading from the windpipe (trachea) to the lungs (Singular: bronchus)

Bronchial   Refers to the bronchi or bronchioles

Bronchial asthma   Allergic asthma. Common form of asthma due to hypersensitivity to an allergen

Bronchial tree   The trachea, bronchi and their branching structures, up to and including the terminal bronchioles

Bronchioles   Smaller subdivisions of the bronchial tubes

Broncho-constriction   Narrowing of the bronchi, usually caused by contraction of the smooth muscles encircling them

Broncho-dilator   Medicine that causes the airways to open

Bronchospasm   Spasm of a bronchus. Sudden or spasmodic bronchoconstriction caused by contraction of the smooth muscles surrounding the airways

Capillaries   Minute, hairlike blood vessels which connect the smallest arteries with the smallest veins

Carbon dioxide   A colorless gas, heavier than air. It is the final metabolic product of carbon compounds present in food. It is eliminated through the lungs

Cardiovascular   Pertains to the heart and blood vessels

Cartilage   A specialized type of dense connective tissue. Found in various parts of the body, including the ribs and the larynx

Catecholamines   Hormones that act on nerve cells

Chronic   Long-term or frequently recurring

Cilia   Hairlike processes projecting from the lining of structures such as the bronchi, which propel mucus, dust particles and other debris

Controller medicine   A medicine that prevents or reduces the frequency and severity of asthma episodes

Corticosteroid   Another term for a steroid or cortisone-like medicine

Cromolyn   Generic name for Intal, a controller medicine that prevents mast cells in the airways from releasing asthma-causing chemicals

Dander   Scales of dead skin

Diaphragm   Dome-shaped muscle of respiration, separating the abdominal and chest cavities, with its convexity upwards. It contracts with each inspiration and relaxes with each expiration. There is also a pelvic diaphragm, which forms the lower boundary of the pelvic cavity

Diuretic   Agent that increases the secretion of urine

DPI   Dry powder inhaler

Dyspnea (also known as Dyspnoea in the UK)   Air hunger resulting in labored or difficult breathing

Endocrine glands   Glands whose secretions (hormones) flow directly into the blood and are circulated to all parts of the body

Enzyme   A complex protein that is capable of inducing chemical changes in other substances without being changed itself

Eosinophils   White blood cells involved in inflammation

Episode (asthma)   Period of time when asthma signs or symptoms occur, peak flow scores drop, breathing is changed, or additional asthma medicine is needed. Sometimes referred to as an 'asthma attack'

Esophagus   Food-pipe. A vital structure essential for carrying foods and liquids from the mouth to the stomach

Exacerbation   Aggravation or increase in severity

Exercise-induced asthma   A form of asthma in which exercise is the only trigger

Expiration   The expulsion of air from the lungs in breathing

Gastroesophageal reflux   Backward flow of material from the stomach to the esophagus. Causes irritation which can lead to bronchospasm

Hemoglobin   The iron-containing pigment of red blood cells. Its function is to carry oxygen from the lungs to the tissues

Histamine   A chemical substance produced when tissues are injured; said to be a factor in causing shock

Holding chamber   Inhalation device used with a metered dose inhaler, which holds the medicine mist to improve its effect

Hormone   A chemical substance which is generated in one organ and carried by the blood to another, in which it excites activity. A secretion of endocrine glands

Hyperventilation   Overbreathing, as occurs in forced respiration. Results in carbon dioxide depletion, with several accompanying symptoms including a fall in blood pressure, anxiety, and sometimes fainting

IgE   Immunoglobulin E, an antibody that reacts with an allergen, initiating the asthma response

Immune system   The body's chief specific defense against disease and other foreign agents. It includes white blood cells, bone marrow, the lymphatic system, the spleen and the thymus gland

Inspiration   Inhalation. Drawing air into the lungs

Intercostal   Between the ribs

Irritant   A non-allergenic substance that may provoke a reaction in the airways

Larynx   The enlarged upper end of the trachea below the root of the tongue. Organ of the voice

Legumes   Fruits or pods of beans, peas or lentils

Leukotriene   Chemical mediator involved in the asthma reaction

Mast cell   One of the cell types that contain chemicals which can produce the asthma reaction

MDI   Metered dose inhaler

Metabolic   Pertains to metabolism

Metabolism   The sum of all physical and chemical changes that take place within an organism

Methacholine challenge   A method of measuring airway activity. It consists of inhaling a saline aerosol as a control, followed by increasing concentrations of methacholine chloride, a substance that slightly narrows the airways, so as to determine their responsiveness. It is used to confirm the diagnosis of asthma when symptoms are present

Metered dose inhaler   Device that creates medicine mist for inhalation, by using a propellant to expel liquid medicine

Mucous membrane   Membrane lining passages and cavities in communication with the air (such as the mouth and nose)

Mucus Viscid fluid secreted by mucous membrane

Nebulizer Apparatus for producing a fine spray or mist

Nedocromil Generic name for Tilade, an anti-inflammatory (controller) medicine

OTC Over the counter. Medicines sold this way do not need a doctor's prescription

Oxidation Process of a substance combining with oxygen

Oxygen A colorless, odorless gas constituting one-fifth of the atmosphere. Essential to respiration

Oxygenate Combine or supply with oxygen

Oxyhemoglobin The combined form of hemoglobin and oxygen. Found in arterial blood. It is the oxygen carrier to body tissues

Peak expiratory flow rate (PEFR) Speed at which air exits the lungs when you give your fastest blast, for a fraction of a second. Also known as peak flow

Peak flow meter A device used to measure peak expiratory flow rate

Pranayama Refers to the integration of the nervous and respiratory systems. Yogic breathing exercises

Prednisolone Oral steroid medicine

Prednisone Generic name of an oral steroid medicine

Pulmonary Concerning or involving the lungs

Pulmonary function test Test or series of tests to measure various aspects of lung function and capacity

RAST Radioallergosorbent test. An allergy test that measures IgE (antibody) to a specific antigen

Respiration Breathing – that is, inspiration and expiration

Respiratory Pertaining to respiration

Retraction 'Sucking in' of the chest or neck skin

Side-effect An undesired or adverse effect of a medicine

Sign   A physical indication (of asthma, for example) that can be noted by an observer

Sinuses   One of the eight bone-enclosed cavities surrounding the nose

Sinusitis   Inflammation of one of the sinuses around the nose

Spacer   A device used with an MDI to improve the effectiveness of a medicine. Also known as a holding chamber or extender

Spirometer   Device used in a doctor's office to measure various components of airflow

Steroid   Type of hormone produced by the cortex (outer layer) of the adrenal glands; has anti-inflammatory properties

Symptoms   Perceptible changes in the body or its functions, which may indicate disease or a phase of disease (such as shortness of breath or tightness of the chest)

Thyroid gland   A two-lobed endocrine gland situated in front of the trachea

Trigger (asthma)   Precipitating factor in causing inflammation of the airways and symptoms of asthma

Wheeze   High-pitched whistling that occurs when air flows through narrowed airways

Bibliography

Adams, Francis V., M.D. *The Asthma Sourcebook* (2nd edn; Los Angeles: Lowell House, 1998)

—. *The Breathing Disorders Sourcebook* (Los Angeles: Lowell House, 1998)

The American Lung Association Advisory Group, with Edelman, Norman H., M.D. *Family Guide to Asthma and Allergies* (Boston: Little Brown and Company, 1997)

American Medical Association. *American Medical Association Essential Guide to Asthma* (New York: Pocket Books, 1998)

Anderson, Kenneth N., Anderson, Lois E., and Glanze, Walter D. (eds). *Mosby's Medical, Nursing & Allied Health Dictionary* (5th edn; St Louis: Mosby-Year Book Inc., 1998)

Balch, Phyllis A., CNC, and Balch, James F., M.D. *Prescription for Nutritional Healing* (3rd edn; New York: Avery, 2000)

Bock, Steven J., M.D., Bock, Kenneth, M.D., and Bruning, Nancy P. *Natural Relief for Your Child's Asthma* (New York: HarperCollins, 1999)

Boutin, Hélène, and Boulet, Louis-Philippe. *Understand and Control Your Asthma* (Montreal & Kingston: McGill-Queen's University Press, 1995)

Brena, Steven. *Yoga & Medicine* (Baltimore: Penguin Books, 1972)

Broadhurst, C. Leigh, Ph.D., with Badmaev, Vladimir, M.D., Ph.D. *The Whole Family Guide to Natural Asthma Relief* (New York: Avery, 2002)

Fanning, Patrick. *Visualization for Change* (Oakland, CA: New Harbinger, 1994)

Fried, Robert, Ph.D. *Breathe Well, Be Well* (New York: John Wiley & Sons, Inc., 1999)

Graham, Judy, and Odent, Dr Michael. *The Z Factor* (Wellingborough, England: Thorsons, 1986)

Greenberg, Alissa, M.D. *Asthma* (New York: Franklin Watts, 2000)

Hendricks, Gay, Ph.D. *Conscious Breathing* (New York: Bantam Books, 1995)

Hogshead, Nancy, and Couzens, Gerald Secor. *Asthma and Exercise* (New York: Henry Holt, 1990)

Horn, Jack C. 'Fighting migraines with The Force', *Psychology Today*, November 1985: page 74

Ivker, Robert S., D.O., and Nelson, Todd, N.D. *Asthma Survival* (New York: Jeremy P. Tarcher/Putnam, 2001)

Kuvalayananda, Swami, and Vinekar, Dr S.L. *Yogic Therapy* (New Delhi: Ministry of Health, Government of India, 1971)

Leigh, Richard, MBChB, MSc, FCPSA, and staff of Firestone Regional Chest and Allergy Unit, St Joseph's Hospital, Hamilton, Ontario, Canada. 'An Overview of Asthma Treatment', *Canadian Respiratory Journal*, March/April 2001, Volume 8, Number 2

Loew, T.H., Tritt, K., Siegfried, W., Bohmann, H., Martus, P., and Hahn, E.G. 'Efficacy of "functional relaxation" in comparison to Terbutaline and a "placebo relaxation" method in patients with acute asthma', *Psychotherapy & Psychosomatics*. 70(3), May–June 2001: pages 151–7

The Merck Manual of Medical Information (Home edition) (New York: Pocket Books, 1997)

Mindell, Earl. *Earl Mindell's Vitamin Bible* (New York: Warner Books, 1979)

Moyers, Bill. *Healing and the Mind* (New York: Doubleday, 1993)

The National Asthma Control Task Force. Report on The Prevention and Management of Asthma in Canada, 2000

Pearce, Evelyn C. *Anatomy and Physiology for Nurses* (13th edn; London: Faber and Faber, 1956)

Plaut, Thomas F., M.D., with Jones, Teresa B., M.A. *Dr Tom Plaut's Asthma Guide for People of All Ages* (Amherst, MA: Pedipress, Inc., 1999)

Rama, Swami, Ballentine, Rudolph, M.D., and Hymes, Alan, M.D. *Science of Breath* (Honesdale, PA: The Himalayan International Institute of Yoga Science and Philosophy, 1979)

Rubin, Bruce K., M.D., and Barnes, Peter J., DM. *Conquering Childhood Asthma* (Hamilton, Ontario, Canada: Empowering Press, 1998)

Silverstein, Alvin, Silverstein, Virginia, and Nunn, Laura Silverstein. *Asthma* (Springfield, NJ: Enslow Publishers, 1997)

Smolley, Lawrence A., M.D., and Bruce, Debra Fulgum. *Breathe Right Now* (New York and London: W.W. Norton & Company, 1998)

Thomas, Clayton L., M.D., M.P.H. (ed.). *Taber's Cyclopedic Medical Dictionary* (15th edn; Philadelphia: F.A. Davis Company, 1985)

Toronto Tuberculosis & Respiratory Disease Association. *So you have Asthma* (1974)

Wechsler, Rob. 'A New Prescription: Mind Over Malady', *Discover*, February 1987: pages 51-61

Weller, Stella. *Yoga in a Box* (London: Thorsons, 2002)

—. *Good Housekeeping Complete Yoga* (London: HarperCollins*Illustrated*, 2001)

—. *The Yoga Back Book* (rev. edn; London: Thorsons, 2000)

—. *The Breath Book* (London: Thorsons, 1999)

—. *Well Being for Women* (New Alresford, UK: Godsfield Press; New York: Sterling, 1999)

—. *Yoga for Children* (London: Thorsons, 1996)

—. *Yoga Therapy* (London: Thorsons, 1995)

—. *Pain-Free Periods* (rev. edn; London: Thorsons, 1993)

—. *Super Natural Immune Power* (Wellingborough, England: Thorsons, 1989)

Wray, Betty B., M.D. *Taking Charge of Asthma* (New York: John Wiley & Sons, 1998)

Yogendra, Smt. Sitadevi. *Yoga Simplified for Women* (Santa Cruz, Bombay: The Yoga Institute, 1972)

Index